Life After Knee Replacement

A Guide to Success with Surgery, Recovery, and Rehabilitation

Life After Knee Replacement

A Guide to Success with Surgery, Recovery, and Rehabilitation

by
Troy A. Miles, MD

Stay active. Live healthy. Get inspired.

Sign up today to get exclusive access to the most authoritative, useful, and cutting-edge information for hip replacement, knee replacement, and shoulder replacement surgery.

Visit us online at www.reddinghipreplacement.com
Join our mailing list at www.reddinghipreplacement.com/join

This book is not a medical manual. The information given here is designed to help you make informed decisions about your health. It is not intended as a substitute for any treatment that you may have been prescribed by your doctor. If you suspect that you have a medical problem, we encourage you to seek competent medical help.

Mention of the specific companies, organizations, or authorities in this book does not imply endorsement by the author or the publisher.
Internet addresses given in this book were accurate at the time it went to print.

© 2017 by Troy A. Miles, MD

This book may be purchased for business or promotional use or for specific sales.

Project Credits
Editor: Stephanie Miles
Illustrations: Septiana Budyastuti
Cover Design: Ilian Georgiev

Manufactured in the United States of America

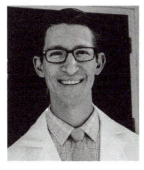

TROY A. MILES, MD is a practicing orthopaedic surgeon in Redding, California, who specializes in the treatment of disorders of the knee, shoulder, and hip, including joint replacement and reconstruction, and arthroscopic surgery. Dr. Miles is a member of the American Association of Hip and Knee Surgeons, American Orthopaedic Association, American Association of Orthopaedic Surgery, and the North Pacific Orthopaedic Society. He has lectured at the Annual Meeting of the North Pacific Orthopaedic Society, the Annual Meeting of the American Society of Surgery of the Hand, and the Annual Meeting of the American Association of Orthopaedic Surgery.

Dr. Miles maintains an active interest in academic medicine, as clinical faculty at UC Davis Medical Center in Sacramento, California.

Author's Note

As you will most likely notice, this book is intended for more than just people experiencing knee pain. My goal in writing Life After Knee Replacement: A Guide to Success with Surgery, Recovery, and Rehabilitation is to provide a comprehensive review of the latest recommendations for both patients and their caregivers.

Oftentimes, well-meaning surgeons will give their patients small brochures and booklets with answers to the most frequently asked questions about knee replacement surgery, but I've found that those educational materials can be very brief with little explanation beyond short statements, and they can gloss over, or miss completely, very important aspects of recovery. I have found that my patients would prefer to have a comprehensive guide that they can refer back to throughout their knee replacement journeys.

My hope is that *Life After Knee Replacement: A Guide to Success with Surgery, Recovery, and Rehabilitation* will become a valuable asset in helping you understand what it is like to have knee replacement surgery and set realistic expectations for your personal recovery process. I've expanded on the material often provided to patients during preoperative clinic appointments with checklists, illustrated guides, and a roadmap for complete recovery after knee replacement surgery.

Troy A. Miles, MD

Contents

Important Note

The material presented in this guide was created to provide a review of information regarding knee replacement surgery. Every effort has been made to offer readers accurate, updated information. The contents of this guide have been compiled through professional research. However, medical professionals have varying opinions and new advances in orthopaedic medicine are made very quickly. As a result, some of the information in this guide may become outdated over time.

The publisher, author, and editors, as well as researchers quoted in this guide, cannot be held responsible for any error, omission, or dated material. Neither the author nor the editors make any warranty, expressed or implied, with respect to the material contained herein. The author assumes no responsibility for any outcome of applying the information in this guide.

If you have any questions concerning the application of the material described in this guide, please consult a qualified surgeon.

Chapter 1
Introduction

If you're like most of the people I see at my practice, your knee pain didn't start yesterday. You have likely been dealing with aches in one or both of your knees for years before deciding to reach out for help. After months to years of debilitating pain that is affecting your general health, mental health, and everyday life, the time has come to seek professional treatment and start feeling better.

Now, it should be noted that this book strictly aims to discuss recovery and rehabilitation after total knee replacement. That means we won't be discussing partial or unicompartmental knee replacement in depth. You might be wondering why that is. Partial knee replacements are performed when only a portion of the knee is damaged by arthritis, and the recovery and functional expectations are much different than that of a total knee replacement.

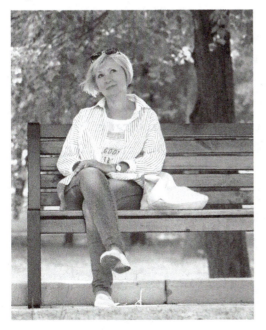

While the details of what it takes to prepare for, undergo, and recover from a significant operation like a knee replacement can feel daunting, I hope to simplify some of the larger aspects of the process so that you can understand what to expect. This guide should also clarify your understanding of what is expected of you during this process, so that you can achieve the best results possible after undergoing total knee replacement surgery.

Knee replacement surgery has some of the highest satisfaction rates amongst orthopaedic procedures. Upwards of 85% to 90% (Noble et al. 2006)(Núñez et al. 2009) of patients who receive knee replacements are very satisfied and say they would have the procedure again. A significant factor in satisfaction following this procedure is knowing what to expect, as well as how to maximize your function and minimize your pain following surgery. (Culliton et al. 2012) In my experience, the greater the understanding patients have about what to expect following knee replacement surgery, the higher the satisfaction. Misunderstandings and a lack of accurate information can lead patients down a path of fear and anxiety, and oftentimes these negative emotions make it harder for people to do the physical work necessary to achieve an optimal result following surgery. Most of my patients have asked questions about the challenges with surgery, recovery and rehabilitation, such as:

1. **Will I be able to play sports again?**
2. **What can I do to make recovery easier?**
3. **When should I be able to drive again?**
4. **How much pain medicine will I need?**
5. **I did a lot of gardening on my hands and knees. Will I be able to kneel?**
6. **Will I need to go to a nursing home after surgery?**
7. **I've heard you can't run after knee replacement. What are other activities I can't do?**
8. **What happens if I walk too much?**
9. **When will my knee be normal again?**
10. **What is the best way to speed up recovery?**

These are only a few of the questions I'm asked every day at my practice; there are too many to list here. The purpose of this guide is to break down the components of a successful recovery and effective rehabilitation following total knee replacement and give you the tools to make this happen. This will require the help and support of your surgeon and his or her team, your therapists, and any loved ones who will be caring for you during the recovery process. While this is ultimately a team effort, there is no substitute for hard work and determination following knee replacement surgery. Achieving your goals following surgery, whatever they may be, is up to you alone.

The decision to proceed with knee replacement surgery should be made in consultation with a board-certified orthopedic surgeon. Your surgeon should discuss your specific condition, as well as options for non-operative treatment, before offering operative intervention as a solution to your knee pain.

Chapter 2
Who Needs a Knee Replacement?

Almost everyone experiences knee pain at some point in life. Common causes for knee pain range from a tear in the ligaments — medial or lateral collateral ligaments, or the anterior or posterior cruciate ligaments — to a tear of the meniscus. Pain also comes from inflammation of the tendons, the patellar or quadriceps tendons, or the hamstring tendons. It can also be due to local areas of cartilage damage, most commonly under the kneecap or one of the condyles of the femur bone. For each of these examples, there are several treatment options available, ranging from non-operative treatments, to operative interventions. However, total knee replacement (TKA) is primarily meant to be the solution if your knee pain is caused by arthritis.

You may ask, "How do I know whether the pain I'm experiencing can be treated with surgery?" The answer is to meet with a physician in person to discuss the symptoms you're experiencing. Based on a thorough evaluation, your provider should be able to tell you:

1) Whether the condition you're experiencing is caused by arthritis.
2) Whether your arthritis can be treated with total knee replacement surgery.
3) Whether you are a good candidate for surgery based on your physical condition, including your general health, mental health, weight, and personal support system.

While there are different forms of arthritis, all of which can be addressed with knee replacement surgery, osteoarthritis is the most common. Osteoarthritis affects upwards of 52.5 million people per year (Hootman et al. 2016). It is characterized by episodic flares of pain, swelling, and stiffness, sometimes without clear causes, which increase in severity and frequency and last longer each episode.

Many forms of inflammatory arthritis, such as rheumatoid arthritis or psoriatic arthritis, are caused by an autoimmune response, which is where your own immune system attacks the cartilage of your joints, wearing it away and eating into the bone itself. Because of recent advancements in medical treatments to suppress the immune system and stop the damage caused to joints, it is becoming increasingly rare for people with inflammatory arthritis to undergo joint replacement surgery. However, in cases where these medical treatments are not effective, and joint disease progresses, knee replacement surgery can still be very beneficial.

Non-Operative Treatment Options

Before considering total knee replacement, you should make sure that you have exhausted all non-operative treatment options. This is for two reasons:

1) There is no reason to subject yourself to the risk and recovery period after a major operation if there are less invasive ways to manage your pain and give you the function you desire.
2) Most insurance companies will not approve and/or pay for surgical intervention unless you have tried, and been unsuccessful with, all non-operative treatments first.

Over-the-Counter Medications

Depending on an individual patient's preference, we will usually begin treatment for knee pain with some type of medication. Over-the-counter medications, which can be used in prescription strength, are the first line of defense against arthritis pain.

If over-the-counter medications aren't helping, then we will move onto prescription formulations of these medications, such as acetaminophen (Tylenol) or ibuprofen (Aleve). Acetaminophen is a non-opioid pain reliever that acts in the brain and masks pain. Acetaminophen does nothing to treat the root cause of the pain, however it can diminish the discomfort. Ibuprofen, and other non-steroidal anti-inflammatory medications, act at the knee joints to reduce inflammation, which is the cause of the pain for people suffering from arthritis. Once again, ibuprofen does not treat the arthritis itself, but it can decrease the painful effects of the arthritis.

Prescription Formulations of Anti-Inflammatories

Over the counter anti-inflammatories (ibuprofen, naproxen, and aspirin) are wonderful medications for arthritis pain relief. They are not without their side effects however. These side effects typically include upset stomach and kidney damage. Several prescription formulations of anti-inflammatories come with fewer side effects. There are also designer anti-inflammatories aimed to block a specific trigger of inflammation, which helps avoid certain side effects. These are called COX-II inhibitors. Finally, gel or ointment formulations of anti-inflammatories can be applied directly to the joint to decrease inflammation. This type of anti-inflammatory medication can be used to help patients avoid upset stomach or kidney damage.

Opioids

If prescription formulations such as as acetaminophen or ibuprofen aren't working, then our next option is to use opioids.

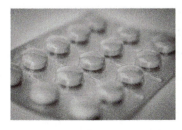

Anti-inflammatories are the best medication for arthritis pain.
These help to minimize the true source of pain, which is inflammation.

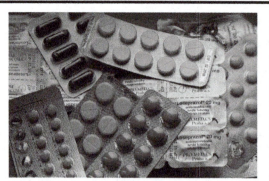

Opioid pain medicine is not an ideal way to manage arthritis pain. *They are not very effective at managing the pain and place you at risk for side effects.*

There has been significant coverage of the current state of opioid use in America, and for good reason. Opioids come with dangerous side effects, the worst being dependence, addiction, and overdose. This is added to the data showing that opioids are not actually very effective at managing arthritis-related pain (da Costa et al. 2014). The longer a patient takes opioid medication, the higher the dose is necessary to achieve the same results. With all of these concerns in mind, it is recommended that people suffering from arthritis not use opioid medications, except for in the most extreme of circumstances. This is especially true given that there are other treatment options available.

The final point to be made regarding opioid pain medication use prior to surgery is that the more you use opioids, the more your body becomes tolerant. As a result, managing your pain following surgery will be more difficult and more risky. Once again, this is because increasing amounts, and stronger types, of opioids are required to ease your pain, which come with increased risk of side effects.

Weight Loss

The next treatment option is weight loss. While not technically considered a form of treatment for knee arthritis, weight loss can have a dramatic, and direct, effect on knee pain. This is due to both the forces on the knee as well as the pro-inflammatory signals that excess body fat produces.

Based on how the knee works during normal gait, the knee sees 1.5 times your bodyweight with every step that you take. This increases to 3 times your bodyweight when climbing stairs or walking up an incline. When you're kneeling or squatting, the knee experiences an incredible 5 times to 7 times your bodyweight. Therefore, for every 1 pound of weight that you lose, your knee will thank you up to 7times.

Osteoarthritis of the knee is an inflammatory disease. This can be made worse if your body is in a proinflammatory state, based on the foods that you eat, medicines that you take, and the amount of body fat that you have. Body fat has been shown to produce signalling molecules that increase your inflammation and activate your immune system (Wisse 2004), which can make existing arthritis more symptomatic and increase progression.

Weight loss also has the effect of decreasing the risk of complications during and after surgery. There has been significant research conducted looking at the association of bodyweight and surgical complications. Based on this data, the American Association of Orthopaedic Surgery recommends undergoing weight management therapy prior to undergoing surgical intervention ("Information Statement" 2016).

Physical Therapy

The next form of treatment is physical therapy. This is a balancing act to increase function while minimizing any additional knee pain caused by the therapy itself. It has been shown that physical activity at least 3 times per week can reduce the risk of arthritis-related disability by 47% (Dunlop et al. 2010). The goal of therapy is to strengthen muscles to decrease forces through painful, arthritic joints, work on proper body mechanics, as well as to instruct the patient on proper use of assistive devices.

Physical therapists can also recommend different treatment options and suggest modifications to your personal environment to make it easier to navigate and decrease painful symptoms.

Steroid Injections

Steroid, or "cortisone", injections are another mainstay of nonoperative treatment for knee arthritis. Injections are available at most medical offices, consisting of some combination of short acting numbing medication, long acting numbing medication, and a steroidal anti-inflammatory medication. Steroids are potent inhibitors of the inflammatory process, and when injected into the area of inflammation, they have a strong effect. Also good news: steroid injections come with minimal side effects, as there is very little absorption into the system at large.

Steroid injections will last varying amounts of time, based on the biology of the patient as well as the state of the knee when the injection is given. As a general rule, injections should not be given any more frequently than once every 3 to 4 months, or 3 to 4 times per year. If injections do not provide adequate relief, or the pain relief does not last long enough in between injections, then they will not be a good treatment option for you in the long term. On the other hand, if steroid injections last longer than 3 to 4 months at a time, and they provide relief allowing you to participate in your desired activities, then they can be used as long as they are effective, sometimes helping people avoid surgery for many years.

Viscosupplementation

Another type of injection for the treatment of knee arthritis is viscosupplementation, or gel/lubrication injections. These are a combination of ground up cartilage and collagen, and synthetic

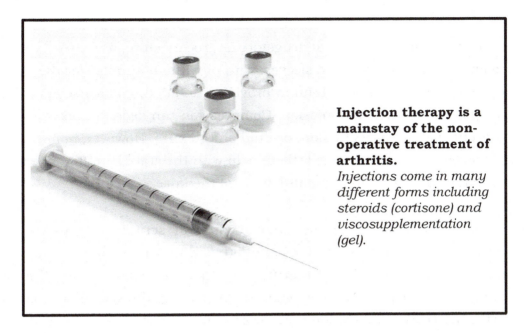

Injection therapy is a mainstay of the non-operative treatment of arthritis.
Injections come in many different forms including steroids (cortisone) and viscosupplementation (gel).

molecules, like chondroitin and glucosamine, which are found in natural cartilage. The idea behind these injections is to provide the building blocks for cartilage while increasing lubrication within the joint, however studies have not proven this to be how viscosupplementation actually works. At this time, there is no clear source of pain relief, and the literature has also not shown viscosupplementation to be significantly more effective than a flip of a coin (Kul-Panza and Berker 2010). Like most treatments in medicine, there are numerous people who get terrific relief from this treatment. And like steroid injections, viscosupplementation may help delay knee replacement surgery for years.

Braces

Bracing is another low risk, potentially high reward non-surgical treatment. While there are several forms of knee braces, they are not created equally. Two general categories of bracing are prescription and non-prescription braces.

Non-prescription, or over the counter, braces are those that are available at any commercial drugstore or grocery store, and they mainly consist of neoprene sleeves, with or without support for the kneecap. These can be helpful in providing an additional sense of support, as well as compression. Compression can decrease and prevent swelling and effusion, or fluid on the knee. However, non-prescription braces do very little to help with the stability of the knee, or to take pressure off of painful areas of the knee.

All prescription braces are not created equal. Prescription braces are designed with specific functions in mind, and they really only work to address a single problem. Unfortunately, there is no single brace that addresses all aspects of knee pain and function in the setting of knee arthritis. The most common type of prescription knee brace is called an unloader brace. An unloader brace is designed to be used in the setting where arthritis primarily affects either the inside or the outside of the knee, with relative maintenance of the opposite portion of the knee. It works to bend the knee away from the affected area, thereby taking pressure off of the painful area of the knee.

To accomplish this, braces have to be large and have significant hardware. They can be bulky, heavy, hot, and they are often very difficult to fit on people's knees. Prescription braces can be pre-fabricated, but these rarely fit well, and they often require custom fitting to each individual's knee anatomy. Even in these scenarios, prescription braces can still have problems after routine wear. For these reasons, they often end up in the closet and not worn.

A good number of patients do find great relief by wearing non-prescription and prescription braces. I've seen a number of patients who were able to forestall surgery for significant periods of time simply by wearing a brace on a daily basis. Regardless of your thoughts on the long-term effectiveness of braces, I still recommend discussing this option with your surgeon before moving onto surgery.

Ambulatory Aids

The final form of non-operative treatment involves ambulatory aids, such as walking sticks, canes, crutches, and walkers. These are less a form of long-term treatment than a necessity once your symptoms of arthritis have become bad enough to limit even the most essential daily functions. Typically, once you get to this point it is time to have a frank discussion with your surgeon regarding surgery.

***

Although less often discussed, it is also important to consider your medical fitness for surgery. Total knee replacement is a major operation, and as such it comes with risk for surgical and postoperative complications. To some extent, complications are unavoidable, meaning you could be the healthiest person in the world and still experience complications. However, if you have pre-existing medical issues, your risks of complications during and after surgery are going to be higher. In order to minimize these risks as much as possible, you should work with your primary care provider to identify any risk factors and come up with a plan to minimize these factors before undergoing surgery.

Common medical conditions that put you at risk for complications are heart disease, diabetes, extremes of body weight, prior history of blood clots, and smoking. If you have any of these issues, it is important to address them before considering surgery. There is an old saying in orthopaedics that there is no problem that surgery cannot make worse. If you have a complication during or after knee replacement surgery, this could not be more true. It is up to you to decrease your risk as much as possible.

Chapter 3

Meeting With Your Surgeon

Once your surgery date is set, you will meet with your surgeon, or someone from his or her team, for a preoperative appointment. This is where you will cross the t's and dot the i's, and ask your additional questions, so there aren't any surprises on the day of your surgery. The last thing you, or your surgeon, wants on the day of surgery is to have to cancel because of a missed medical issue or unforeseen circumstance.

The surgeon will review your blood work, re-examine your knee, and inspect your leg for any cuts, rashes, or sores during this final pre-operative appointment. The surgeon will also review the surgery to the detail that you desire and complete a consent form with you. He will have you sign this form and confirm the final details for the day of surgery. Included on this consent form will typically be instructions, such as when to stop eating and drinking before surgery, where to show up, what to bring with you, and how long your hospital stay is expected to be.

Before leaving your preoperative appointment, be sure to ask about a prescription for postoperative pain medicine, along with the medicine you will use for blood thinning and any orthotic devices, such as knee braces,

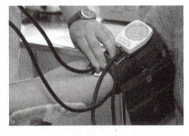

Expect to be checked in by several teams in the pre-operative area. You will be seen by your surgeon's team, the anesthesia team, and two nursing teams to ensure that you are prepared for surgery.

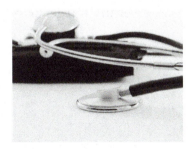

Once the check in process is complete, you will head to the OR. In the operating room, you will undergo anesthesia, have additional IV lines placed, and be positioned on the operating table for surgery.

29

walkers, and compression stockings. Most surgeons will prescribe medications during the final preoperative appointments to give patients time to gather the necessary supplies before the day of surgery.

The following is a checklist of questions you should make sure to ask your surgeon.

- ❏ Pre-op x-rays: Have they been done?
- ❏ Pre-op labs: Were there any abnormalities?
- ❏ Pain medicine: Was it prescribed, and how should it be taken?
- ❏ Blood thinners: Was it prescribed and how should it be taken?
- ❏ Walker: Was it prescribed and how should it be used?
- ❏ Brace: Was it prescribed and how should it be used?
- ❏ Compression stockings: Was it prescribed and how should it be used?
- ❏ What can I do to decrease my risk of infection following surgery?
- ❏ What will my discharge destination be?
- ❏ Length of stay: What is the anticipated length of stay after surgery?
- ❏ Follow up appointments: When should I see the surgeon again after my surgery?

Chapter 4
Preparing For Surgery Day

Planning for the day of your surgery is absolutely critical. Once you have exhausted all of your non-operative options, you have optimized your general health, and you have come to the conclusion that knee replacement surgery is the right decision for you, the next step in your journey will be to schedule and prepare for your knee replacement surgery. Although your surgeon and medical care team will play a key role on this important day, there are also things that you can do as the patient to make the recovery process after surgery as easy and successful as possible. In order to understand how you should prepare for your surgery day, become familiar with these four areas of focus.

1. Preparing the Home

Preparing your home before surgery day is a key component to a successful, complication-free recovery.

Recovery Zones

A safe recovery zone is where you will spend the majority of your early time after surgery. This recovery zone is where you should store the majority of the items that you may need at any given time.

Everyone's recovery zone will look different, but this should universally be an area that provides a comfortable place to sit, rest, and even possibly sleep. The recovery zone should also have easy access to water, a pain pill or two, a small snack, television remotes, a telephone or communication device, and reading material. The ultimate goal is to create a safe space where everything is accessible, so that you do not need to get up frequently in the early period of your recovery.

Most patients who have recently undergone knee replacement surgery find that the most comfortable place to sleep is on a recliner chair or a sectional sofa.

In addition, it is prudent to arrange your environment to aid in mobility and clear your home of obstacles and impediments that may act as tripping hazards. Common tripping hazards include cords, wires, loose rugs, dogs, cats, shoes, purses or bags, low side tables or coffee tables, and door thresholds.

Ideally, your recovery zone will be close to a restroom, and it will also be close to the place where you will sleep at night. (This is not necessarily the bedroom, as we will discuss later in this chapter.) Although you will want to get up and take short walks about your home at least every couple of hours, you do not want to have to walk significant distances, or go up stairs, to get to your bedroom or restroom.

Identifying Tripping Hazards

The next aspect of preparing your home is identifying potential tripping hazards and finding ways to minimize the risk that these items present. Common tripping hazards include loose rugs, power cords, coffee tables, and raised door thresholds between rooms. Items that are easily moved should be taken out of the recovery zone, so as to not get in the way when you are up and about.

Clearing loose debris and cleaning your entryways can also decrease the risk of slipping and falling after surgery. Depending on when your surgery takes place, there may be leaves or other debris about your entryway. This can easily be overlooked, however it should be addressed, as you will be using your entryway when you are coming from and going to physical therapy appointments.

Of course, some aspects of the home are not modifiable. For example, it's tough to move a door threshold. Any tripping hazards that cannot be moved or modified should be marked clearly, so that they are easy to see while walking. This is important, even if you have lived in your home for years. After surgery, you will be taking pain medications, recovering from anesthesia, and likely very fatigued from surgery itself, all of which make it easy to forget the details of your surroundings.

Preparing the Bathroom

Finally, preparing your bathroom is an important consideration before surgery. Depending on your bathroom arrangement, you may not need additional modifications to make it easier for you to navigate. It can be helpful, however, to make sure that you have something sturdy to grab onto and use to rise from the toilet, as well as while getting into and out of the shower. You may want to consider installing hand rails around the toilet and inside the shower. These can be temporary in nature, or more permanent, depending on the type of product you choose. Shower seats are also an aid that is very important in the early days and weeks following knee replacement surgery. In most cases, handrails, shower seats, and other bathroom modification devices are very helpful in preventing falls.

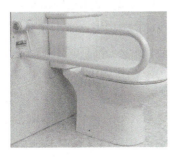

Bathroom modifications should be made before surgery takes place.
Hand rails or grab bars make it easier to use the restroom safely following surgery.

2. Pre-Hab

Physical therapy plays a major role in recovery from knee replacement surgery. A large part of your satisfaction level after knee replacement will involve the range of motion in your knee. The more range of motion you can achieve following surgery, the happier you're likely to be with the outcome. Increased range of motion happens through hard work and determination with your therapist. While physical therapy following knee replacement is not an easy process, mainly because of the timing of therapy following a major surgery, there are things that you can do to make it easier on yourself. This includes pre-hab.

The term "pre-hab" can mean one of several things, depending on the definition that your surgeon uses. Some surgeons will have their patients visit a physical therapist once before surgery to establish a connection and review certain exercises, and expectations, for postoperative therapy prior to surgery. Other surgeons will take a different approach, having their patients participate in specific preoperative therapy programs for a number of weeks to strengthen the muscles around the knee and maximize the knee range of motion prior to surgery.

This is based on the idea that your quadricep muscles play a very important role in your recovery and satisfaction with knee replacement surgery. These muscles are often weak heading into surgery due to favoring one leg over the other because of the knee pain. This is made worse by surgery itself, which traumatizes the quadriceps muscle. Recovery of this muscle plays a large role in your symptoms following surgery, as your knee motion will not be smooth and "normal" until this muscle regains its strength. Regaining that strength can take months, or even up to a year post-surgery. Good evidence shows that strengthening the quadriceps muscle can minimize symptoms such as knee and quad soreness, developing fluid on your knee, and strain of the ligaments on the sides of your knee, and it may shorten the duration of time that you experience these symptoms at all. (Skoffer et al. 2016)

Good evidence also exists showing that the final range of motion of your knee after surgery is closely related to the degree of motion before surgery. (Ritter et al. 2004) Researchers have shown that patients can increase their range of motion with physical therapy before surgery even takes places. (Deyle et al. 2000) Based on this evidence, I have started recommending that many of my patients participate in formal physical therapy programs prior to knee replacement in order to improve their results following surgery.

Not every surgeon shares the same opinion regarding pre-hab recommendations, however it is a good idea to bring up the topic with your provider during an initial clinical appointment. In some cases, there may be issues with insurance coverage for pre-operative therapy, either due to clinical necessity or because some insurance carriers are limiting the number of paid visits following surgery, however this depends largely on the insurance policy and it is best discussed with your personal surgeon and insurance company directly.

3. Support Systems

Recovery from knee replacement surgery is not a solo journey. Make sure to have people around you who will be there when you need an extra boost or pick-me-up following surgery. You'll also need people who you can call and count on in the event that you need someone to be physically there for you. For many people, this is not a difficult requirement to meet, but for others, finding a support system for the early weeks following surgery is not so easy.

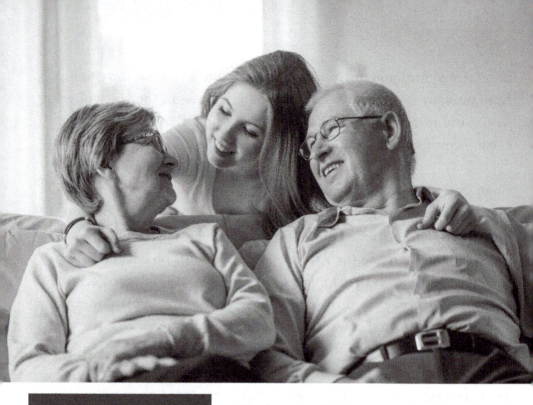

Having a reliable support system is extremely important, as there is good evidence to support going home as opposed to going to a nursing or rehabilitation facility after surgery. Patients who return to their own homes do tend to have better results. Going to a nursing facility or rehabilitation hospital is associated with increased risk of adverse events for both primary (first time) and revision (re-do) patients. (Keswani, Weiser, et al. 2016) Patients who go to a nursing facility or rehabilitation hospital following total knee replacement are statistically more likely to experience falls, infection, or a return to the emergency department during the early weeks after surgery. Although there is not a clear consensus within the medical community as to why this occurs, there is good data to show that this is the case.

4. Healthy Diet

The final area of preparation prior to surgery is establishing a healthy diet to provide your body with the necessary building blocks to heal your wounds, build muscle for recovery and proper knee function, and support your immune system. Surgery is a large stress on your body which requires significant healing to occur, it is important to set yourself up for success.

Poor nutrition before surgery has been shown to increase the risk of complications. (Walls et al. 2015) The most serious complications that can result from malnutrition are wound healing issues and infection. Malnutrition can also delay recovery, as it is impossible to build muscle and strength without the adequate nutritional building blocks.

Maintaining a healthy diet prior to surgery is no more complicated than what your mother told you as a child. Eat your greens and lean meats, and stay away from the junk foods. This means limiting any carbohydrates, refined sugars, and processed foods, and focusing instead on eating fruits, vegetables, chicken, and fish.

While there are any number of different diets and strategies that can help patients improve their nutrition status leading up to surgery, there are several common traits among the most successful diet plans. These are frequent small meals, a focus on foods that are high in protein and fiber, staying well hydrated, and avoiding fried foods, fatty meats, and processed foods.

On the following page you will see a handout developed in association with the nutrition department at Oregon Health & Science University and based upon the "Healthy Eating Plate" from the Harvard Medical School and Harvard School of Public Health. Although every patient should take steps to improve his or her nutrition prior to surgery, the specifics of any plan should be discussed personally with your surgeon.

Your surgeon may also specifically order laboratory tests to evaluate your nutrition, and depending on the results, he or she may recommend a nutritionist leading up to surgery.

Pre-Surgery Diet

Don't skip meals. Eat within one hour of waking, then have a meal or snack every three to four waking hours.

Include lean protein and a high-fiber food (such as fruit, vegetables or a whole grain) at all meals and snacks.

Aim for 64 ounces of fluids daily in order to stay hydrated; choose water or other calorie-free beverages.

Use the "Healthy Eating Plate" below to create balanced, nutritious meals. Avoid fried foods, fatty meats, and processed foods.

Snack ideas:
- ▶ Greek yogurt & fruit
- ▶ Small handful of nuts and dried fruit
- ▶ Hummus and veggies
- ▶ Low-fat cheese & four whole grain crackers
- ▶ Peanut butter or almond butter with apple slices

Healthy Eating Plate

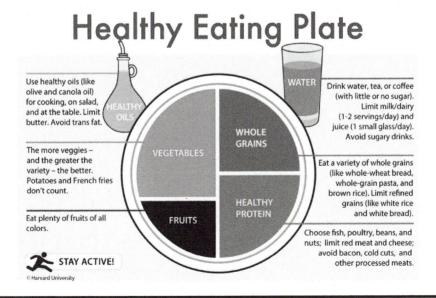

Use healthy oils (like olive and canola oil) for cooking, on salad, and at the table. Limit butter. Avoid trans fat.

The more veggies – and the greater the variety – the better. Potatoes and French fries don't count.

Eat plenty of fruits of all colors.

STAY ACTIVE!

© Harvard University

Drink water, tea, or coffee (with little or no sugar). Limit milk/dairy (1-2 servings/day) and juice (1 small glass/day). Avoid sugary drinks.

Eat a variety of whole grains (like whole-wheat bread, whole-grain pasta, and brown rice). Limit refined grains (like white rice and white bread).

Choose fish, poultry, beans, and nuts; limit red meat and cheese; avoid bacon, cold cuts, and other processed meats.

WATER

HEALTHY OILS

VEGETABLES

WHOLE GRAINS

FRUITS

HEALTHY PROTEIN

Chapter 5

Surgical Treatment Plans

When most people think about knee replacement, they focus on the surgery itself. But patients who've gone through the process before, and those who researched what to expect by reading books like this, know that the real changes happen outside the operating room. By coming up with a comprehensive treatment plan prior to the day of surgery, patients and their providers can be clear about expectations, potential pitfalls, and best practices to ensure an optimal result.

Knee replacement surgery and recovery is not a solo journey. In addition to the support you will receive from your close circle of friends and family, you will work together with a team of healthcare professionals. In this section, we will discuss the process of working with your healthcare team and the appointments you will have leading up to and following surgery.

1. Pre-Surgery Office Visits

Every knee replacement surgery starts with a simple office visit. Depending on the practice of your surgeon, this initial visit may be completed by a physician assistant or a nurse practitioner. Meeting with a physician assistant or nurse practitioner in lieu of the surgeon is very common, and it allows your surgeon to spend more time discussing the operation itself with patients who qualify for surgery. The initial visit at your surgeon's office is very much a screening

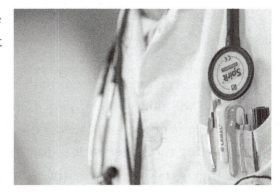

visit. During this visit, the health care practitioner is looking to see that:

A.You have a problem that the surgeon can address
B.You have already tried all non-operative treatment options, or understand why they might not apply to you
C.You are interested in pursuing surgical treatment to address your problem

The referral process to a surgeon's office is not perfect, and oftentimes patients come into the office with problems that cannot be addressed through knee replacement surgery. For example, someone who has a torn ligament or meniscus, but presents with with very little arthritis, is unlikely to be a good candidate for knee replacement surgery. A person in this condition would be better off seeing an orthopaedic sports medicine specialist who focuses on treating these types of injuries.

After it has been established that severe knee arthritis is the source of your symptoms, that you have exhausted all of your non-surgical options, and that you are interested in moving forward with knee replacement surgery, then you will meet with the surgeon who will be performing your procedure. Once again, depending on the surgeon's individual practice, he may meet with you at the time of your initial evaluation or he may have you return for a separate evaluation to focus more specifically on surgery itself.

Once the decision has been made to proceed with surgery, your surgeon will notify his surgery scheduler and initiate the process of getting your operation date on the books. This begins with completing the paperwork to justify to your insurance company that this is the correct treatment for the correct diagnosis.

This process varies in length depending on the insurance carrier, but can sometimes take weeks to complete. Once approval has been granted by the insurance carrier, then the surgery scheduler will contact you about potential surgical dates.

Medical Clearances Before Surgery

Most joint replacement surgeons will require pre-surgical clearance from a primary care provider or specialized pre-operative clinic prior to scheduling surgery. Some surgeons may also require more specialized pre-surgical examinations, such as a visit to the cardiologist, even for patients who do not have a history of heart problems. Knee replacement surgery places stress on the heart and lungs, and it can expose underlying issues that may not have been identified previously. A cardiologist will run routine tests to hopefully prevent this from happening.

Many surgeons will also have you evaluated by a licensed dentist to be sure that you do not have any dental infections or need invasive dental work prior to surgery. The reason behind this recommendation is because dental infections and invasive dental work can increase the risk for infection in the replaces knee. As a result, these issues need to be addressed prior to proceeding with surgery. Most joint replacement centers have informational classes

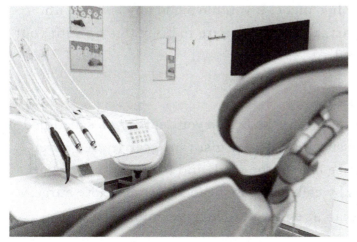

where team members will review the pre-surgery process with patients. This is your best opportunity to meet the nurses and therapists who will be caring for you in the hospital. It will also be a good opportunity to ask any questions that you may have about what to expect before, after, or during your surgery.

Final Pre-Operative Appointments

Between one and two weeks before the date of your surgery, your surgeon or his physician's assistant will likely ask to see you back in the clinic for a final pre-operative appointment. The goal for this pre-operative appointment is for the medical team to complete a final review and ask any last-minute questions to ensure there will not be any surprises on the day of surgery. Remember, the surgical clearance evaluation your primary care doctor, cardiologist, and dentist were asked to complete? Well, this appointment is the time when those evaluation will be reviewed. It's likely that you will be asked to submit a final blood and urine test at this appointment, as well.

The final pre-operative appointment is the last chance to address any issues, and verify any non-routine aspects of your medicall care before proceeding with the knee replacement surgery. An example of some of the non-routine aspects of care that your medical team may be looking at include allergies to specific medications, blood thinners, or recommendations that your primary care doctor has made. If you have had any issues with anesthesia in the past, please make sure to bring this up with your medical team, as well.

Insurance Verification

During the last one to two weeks before your surgery is scheduled to take place, make sure to call your insurance carrier. It's never fun to receive surprise bills in the mail, and the best way to avoid unexpected costs is by calling the insurance carrier before surgery and asking to speak to a representative. I recommend asking specifically about the process of knee replacement surgery from their end, including a review of çoverage and an estimate of your personal expenses. Although these will be general numbers, they should give you a better idea of what your expected contribution will be. For some, hearing these numbers may provoke a certain amount of anxiety, but for many others it is comforting to have the knowledge of what type of bills to expect in the weeks and months following surgery. Establishing contact with your insurance company prior to surgery can also give you a leg up if you need to make contact again after surgery is complete, such as if you are calling to dispute a claim or to make sure that a billing mistake has not been made.

2. Surgery Day

Expect to arrive two to three hours prior to your scheduled operation time on the day of surgery. This will allow the medical team time to get you checked in and fully prepared for surgery. The analogy I like best has to do with air travel. It does not matter if you are flying somewhere local or across the globe, the process for checking-in— dropping off your bags, boarding the plane, finding your seat, etcetera — is very much the same as it is for surgery, as well.

Regardless of how much paperwork it seems like you've gotten at previous office visits, expect to have even more forms to fill out on the day of surgery. Once the paperwork is completed, you will be taken to the pre-surgery area and asked to change into your hospital gown, and a nurse will review your records, which include a medical history, the reason for the surgery, and any allergies or medications you are currently on. At this point, the nurse will start an IV line and begin giving you some pre-medications.

One of the ways we avoid medical mistakes is by verifying the side and site of every patient's knee replacement prior to surgery. Expect your surgeon or his assistant to come in once your IV line has been started to place his or her initials at the correct site on your skin. This is also a good time to ask any last-minute questions you may have. You will meet with the anesthesia doctor, who will explain his or her role in the procedure and review what options you may have for pain relief and sedation.

If this seems like a lot, that's because it is. We take every precaution to make surgery as safe as possible for patients, and seeing these steps listed out can be overwhelming. But, these steps tend to happen seamlessly once you arrive at the surgery center on the day of your procedure, and there is very little you need to do other than to relax and answer any questions from the medical team.

When it is time for your operation to begin, you will say goodbye to your loved ones and be rolled on a gurney into the operating room. You will then be transferred to the operating table and placed in the appropriate position for anesthesia.

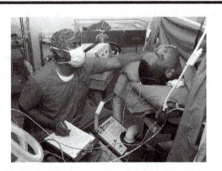

To Sleep or Not to Sleep?
Several different options are available for anesthesia during your operation. The current trend is to have a spinal block. Similar to epidural injections used in child birth, a spinal block numbs the legs only, avoiding the need for powerful medications that turn off the brain. A spinal block can be coupled with sedation, which can make you as sleepy as you prefer to be.

A spinal block is different than "going to sleep," otherwise known as general anesthesia. General anesthesia involves a breathing tube, while a spinal block allows you to breath on your own. This minimizes several of the side effects of general anesthesia, which include nausea and stress on the heart, lungs, and brain. General anesthesia can also slow down your ability to participate in rehabilitate after surgery.

Anesthesia Options
A quick note regarding anesthesia: There are many options for pain relief and sedation during surgery, and no single approach is right for everyone. With that being said, it has been generally accepted in the last 10 to 20 years that knee replacement surgeries work best when they are done under a spinal block with varying levels of sedation.

A spinal block involves receiving a single injection of numbing medication into the lower back, which blocks the nerves below the waist. However, spinal blocks are not an option for everyone. Specifically, if you have had prior low back surgery or have severe low back arthritis, it can be difficult or impossible for the anesthesiologist to get the medication into the right place. For those who are good candidates for spinal blocks, this is truly a better option than the standard "general" anesthesia for several reasons:

A spinal block tends to work better than general anesthesia for patients undergoing knee replacement surgery because it creates less stress on the heart, lungs, bowels, and other internal organs, and it does not affect the brain. A spinal block also has less of an affect on memory loss, haziness, and delirium, and it comes with fewer side effects, such as nausea and vomiting. Patients who opt for spinal blocks are able to get up and participate in physical therapy much more quickly than those who undergo general anesthesia, which decreases the risk of bed sores, blood clots, and bowel obstruction. Simply speaking, spinal blocks provide better pain control, requiring fewer pain medications, which also come with downsides and side effects. (Horlocker et al. 2006)

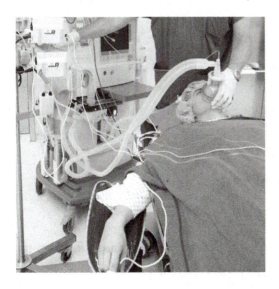

Having said all of this, if previous surgeries or other concerns limit your options and you need to have general anesthesia, it does not mean that you will not recover well. There are still a number of surgeons who recommend general anesthesia for all knee replacement surgeries, and many of these surgeons have great outcomes. General anesthesia has a long track record, however it does come with some additional side effects that should be taken into consideration.

If you are having general anesthesia, you will be placed on your back in a comfortable position, and your anesthesia doctor will give you an oxygen mask to breathe. Once you have taken several deep breaths of oxygen, the doctor will give you the medication and you will be off to sleep before you even realize it.

If you undergo a spinal block you will sit on the operating table like a park bench. The anesthesia doctor will instruct you further on putting yourself in the correct position depending on your size and stature, but it will likely be a slouched position that pushes your low back out toward the doctor. A spinal block is typically done after you have received some relaxation medication to take the edge off, since getting an injection while sitting in the operating room and preparing to have major surgery can be nerve wracking. Rest assured that your surgeon and every member of the medical team will be doing everything they can to make the process as comfortable and stress-free as possible.

Expect to be positioned on your back and placed on the operating table once your spinal block is complete. Your surgeon and his team will then begin placing several devices and other positioners to monitor your vitals signs, secure you to the table, pad your arms and legs, squeeze your non-operative leg to keep blood flowing and prevent blood clots, and keep you warm.

Expectations During Surgery
Once you are in the correct position for surgery, it is time to prepare your skin. This can be done in one of several ways, which your

surgeon will decide based on his training and current evidence for effective cleaning solutions and techniques. Some surgeons prefer cleaning the leg with a combination of alcohol solution, iodine solution, and chlorhexidine soap solution.

Skin cleansing is very important due to the fact that we always have bacteria covering our skin. Normally these bacteria do not cause any problems, and can be beneficial by preventing bad bacteria from setting up residence and causing infections. In the setting of surgery, these normal bacteria can gain access to your wound and cause infections. For this reason, we try to rid your skin of as many of these bacteria as we possibly can to minimize or eliminate this risk.

Surgical drapes will go up once the skin has been thoroughly cleansed. In these last few moments before surgery begins, the entire medical team will take a "time out" to verify your identity, surgical site, and the details of your procedure. Everyone in the room will discuss the important details of the surgery and the post-surgery care plan, including any allergies and antibiotics given, to prevent medical errors. When everyone in the room is in agreement, the surgeon will begin the procedure.

Total knee replacement surgery can last anywhere from 45 to 90 minutes, depending on the technical details of the patient's knee and the surgeon's technique. If you are interested in the actual steps of the procedure, there are several videos available on the internet. I would caution, however, that these types of surgical videos can be quite explicit, and you may want to skip watching any if you have an aversion to blood or other surgical images.

3. Post-Surgery

As your surgery concludes, the surgeon will close your wound, bandages will be applied, and the surgical drapes will be taken down.

You will then be transferred to the postanesthesia care unit for observation while your anesthesia wears off. Depending on the type of anesthesia you received, this part of the process can take anywhere from 30 minutes to a few hours. Once you are alert and awake enough to converse, your family members will be invited back to see you.

From the postanesthesia care unit, you will be transferred to a more typical hospital room. This is where you're likely to meet the nurse and others members of the team that will be caring for you and providing you with assistance in all activities during your hospital stay. Depending on your surgeon's protocol, you may also meet your physical therapists and get out of bed for the first time shortly after arriving in your hospital room.

While rest is not easy to come by in a hospital, it is an extremely important part of recovery and rehabilitation from knee replacement surgery.

Now it's time to rest, relax, and truly begin therecovery process. Your energy stores will already be depleted significantly, as so much of your reserves are being devoted to healing the large "injury" that was created by surgery. In light of this, you need to do everything possible to maximize your energy in order to participate more fully in physical therapy.

Over the next one to two days, you will work with physical therapy on getting in and out of bed, getting up to a chair and the restroom, walking a distance with a walker (typically 100 feet), and getting into and out of a car, as well as going up and down a few stairs. Once you have demonstrated an understanding and ability to accomplish these goals, you will be cleared by your therapist to return home.

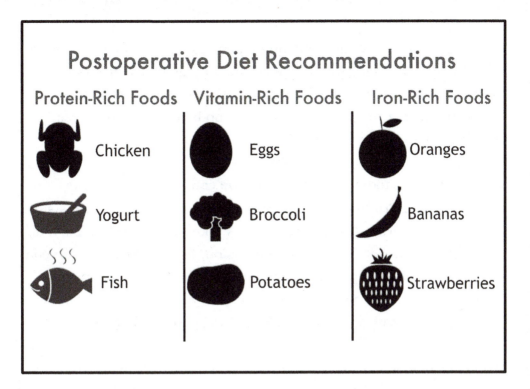

Postoperative Diet Recommendations

Protein-Rich Foods	Vitamin-Rich Foods	Iron-Rich Foods
Chicken	Eggs	Oranges
Yogurt	Broccoli	Bananas
Fish	Potatoes	Strawberries

Diet After Surgery

With the "injury" from surgery, anesthesia, and slow bowel function, which is affected by surgery, along with pain medications and immobility, you may have a decreased appetite. While force feeding is certainly not necessary, it is important to have something to eat at every meal, and snacks in between to help keep your energy up.

It may take days before your bowels begin functioning at full capacity following surgery, and eating too much too soon can overload them and cause nausea, vomiting, or worse yet, a bowel blockage, which can significantly complicate recovery. Luckily, this is a rare occurrence. When it comes to a post-surgery diet, most people will be fine when they follow their own hunger cues.

Pain Control

Your pain also needs to be under control before you'll be cleared to return home after surgery. Pain control is very important after total knee replacement. Without adequate pain control, a patient's ability to participate in therapy is limited. Pain can also have effects on general health. Poor pain control may increase a patient's blood pressure, heart rate, and put his or her body in a state of stress, which ultimately slows down the recovery process.

On the flip side, too much pain medicine can also have serious consequences. Traditional pain medicine comes with numerous side effects ranging from simple annoyances, like itching and nausea, to fatal side effects, like breathing depression. For this reason, surgeons often try to only give patients the amount of pain medication they need — and nothing more. As surgeons, we also try to attack pain from different angles with multiple types of pain medications.

Pain control following knee replacement is an area of very active and extensive research. There has been a shift toward using a multimodal approach to postoperative pain control in the last decade. This includes different types of medications to address the different sources of pain, timing of medications, and specialized anesthesia techniques before, during, and after surgery for controlling pain and numbing the knee.

Surgeons can't take a one-size-fits-all approach to pain management because the pain that patients experience following total knee replacement comes from a number of different sources. During the first few days following surgery, pain may be caused by tissue damage, inflammation, nerve irritation, and swelling, among other factors. To address each of these sources, I recommend providing patients with medications aimed specifically at each source of pain. A few examples of the different medication groups we have available are traditional opioid pain medications (such as oxycodone), anti-inflammatories (such as ketorolac), and nerve stabilizers (such as gabapentin). Surgeons may also recommend non-medicinal treatments like cold therapy, body positioning supports, and assistive devices to limit additional stress during the early phase of recovery.

Medication timing also plays an important role in helping to minimize pain following knee replacement. Pain control starts with pre-medication before surgery even begins. A pre-medication regimen may include all of the medications previously discussed in this section, along with special nerve blocks performed by an anesthesiologist before surgery begins. Nerve blocks are injections of numbing medication directly targeting the nerves that provide sensation to the areas in and around the knee joint. The idea behind this is that pain activates certain parts of the body's nervous system and brain, and if we can prevent these areas from being activated before a patient is in pain, then we can effectively decrease the overall level of discomfort after surgery.

Pain control following knee replacement is an important aspect of recovery, but it can be challenging to manage pain for patients who have been taking opioid medications prior to surgery. Once the body has been exposed to pain medications, it develops a tolerance and more medication is needed in order to achieve the same level of pain control.

As you take more medication to control your pain after knee replacement, the risk of serious complications increases. For this reason, it is very important to work with your surgeon and the physician prescribing these medications to try and wean from the medications as much as possible leading up to surgery. Your surgeon may also suggest that you see a pain medicine specialist to help in this weaning process. A pain medicine specialist may be able to recommend strategies for managing pain following surgery, as well.

With all medications come side effects. The most consistent side effect of opioid pain medication is constipation. Inflammation from the surgery, the effects of anesthesia, and the relatively inactive state that patients are in following surgery also play a role in constipation after surgery. To help decrease constipation, patients are typically given a combination of softening and bowel activating medications following knee replacement surgery.

Based on your surgeon's specific protocol, there are several other medications that you may receive during your hospital stay. Please discuss these medication options with your surgeon prior to your surgery day.

Returning Home

The amount of time you spend in the hospital may vary depending on the philosophy of your surgeon and care team. Many surgeons were taught that it is good to keep patients in the hospital, so they can be observed and treated immediately if anything goes awry during the first few days after surgery. The flip side, however, is that staying in the hospital may increase the chances of a patient suffering an infection after surgery. Longer hospital stays may also be associated with higher rates of blood clots, pneumonia, falls, and an overall lack of sleep, which slows the recovery process. Unless you have to be there for medical reasons, it is usually better to recover from knee replacement surgery in the comfort and familiar environment of your own home.

Most patients in the United States return home from the hospital two to three days following total knee replacement surgery, but this can vary depending on the patient's location. A growing number of surgical centers are making an effort to get people home on the same day as their surgeries, or the first day after. While there are still many facilities that have patients staying upwards of seven days following surgery, the general trend seems to be toward shorter lengths of stay following total knee replacement. This is due in large part to the significant amount of research and data that's now available showing the benefits of returning home earlier following knee replacement surgery. (Barad, Howell, and Joyce 2015)

Recent evidence shows that being discharged to a nursing or rehabilitation facility following knee replacement surgery leads to increased risk of everything from heart attack and blood clots, to falls and pneumonia. The likelihood of readmission to the hospital is increased, as well, compared to those that went home directly from the hospital. (Keswani, Tasi, et al. 2016) Of course, researchers have only analyzed the numbers, and they have not yet offered a potential reason for why it may be more dangerous for patients to stay in nursing or rehabilitation facilities following surgery. Some have hypothesized that this is likely due to being in a foreign environment, not being comfortable with the care team, and being exposed to things like infections and increased stress.

For this reason, in my practice I strongly encourage patients to arrange for help at home even if this means that a family member has to fly in after surgery. In cases where a stay at a rehabilitation facility following total knee replacement cannot be avoided, we take every precaution to avoid complications.

Chapter 6

Avoiding Post-Surgery Complications

All surgeries come with risk of complications, and unfortunately total knee replacement is no exception. Overall, total knee replacement is an incredibly safe and beneficial surgery, and there are ways to minimize the risks as much as possible. Here are some of the most common complications, along with information about how to avoid them.

1. Blood Clots

Blood clots in the deep veins of the legs can be a serious complication after surgery. Thankfully, this is a potential complication that surgeons are well aware of, and it is something they spend time working to prevent.

Common signs of blood clots in the leg are increased swelling, increased tenderness in the calf or thigh, or a change in color of the leg — to purple, blue, or sometimes even bright red. When a blood clot occurs, there is usually a change in pain level, and current medication dosages no longer feel like they're working quite as well. If

you experience these symptoms, alert your surgeon or go to the emergency room right away.

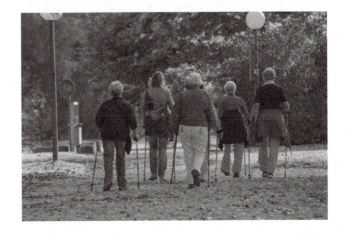

We can prevent blood clots from occurring in several ways, starting with the way patients are positioned in the operating room.

Placing a calf squeezer on the leg that is not having the knee replacement keeps the blood flowing through your veins to prevent stasis, which can lead to blood clots. After surgery is complete, the surgical leg will also have a calf pump placed. These pumps are hooked to an air machine, which periodically pumps up the squeezers on the legs and forces the blood in the veins back to the heart. These devices should be on and working anytime the patient is in bed. If they are not on, please take the initiative to inform your nurse and have them replaced.

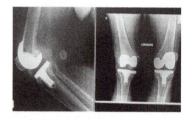

X-rays are a routine method for monitoring knee implants.
You will have x-rays taken after your surgery, while you are in the hospital. You will then have another set of x-rays taken of your new knee replacement approximately six weeks after surgery.

Blood thinning medications can also reduce instances of blood clots after surgery. This is another area of active research within the orthopaedic surgery community. Several types of blood thinning medication exist, from simple "low power" medications like aspirin, to very strong ones, like coumadin/warfarin, which require you to have blood drawn several times per week to ensure that your blood is not too thin. Depending on your personal risk factors, your surgeon may recommend one of the many other blood thinning medications currently on the market. Regardless of the specific type of blood thinner your surgeon recommends, it is important to take the medication diligently.

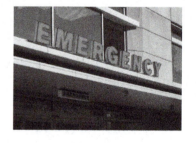

If you have any concerns after being discharged from the hospital, always call your surgeon's office.
You should have clear contact information for your surgeon's team in the event that you have any concerns after returning home. If you experience a true emergency, proceed directly to your nearest emergency department and instruct the staff to inform your surgeon immediately,

Blood thinners should be started within 24 hours of the operation, and you should continue taking the medication for the next two to four weeks, if not longer. As these medications make bleeding more likely, it is important to monitor yourself and watch for any signs of excess blood loss. If you notice blood loss around the surgical area, or if you begin to feel faint, light headed, dizzy when standing up, short of breath, or like you are having heart palpitations, it may be a sign that you are losing too much blood and you should alert your care team right away. Thankfully, this is a rare event.

The last, and possibly most important, strategy for preventing blood clots is also the most simple — getting out of bed and moving around. Movement is the natural way to keep blood flowing through the legs, which the calf pumps try to recreate. The more often you are able to get up and move, the more effective this is. Keep in mind, you don't have to do much for movement to be effective. Something as simple as standing up and changing the chair you are sitting in can help.

2. Infection

Infection is one of the worst things that can happen after a total knee replacement. To have an infection is a life changing event, somewhat analogous to developing cancer. This is true both in treatment as well as prognosis.

Unless the infection is superficial and limited only to the outer portions of the skin, treatment of an infected total knee replacement will typically involve a year-long journey that begins with one to two "clean out" surgeries. During these surgeries, it is likely that the knee implant will need to be removed.

Taking out a knee replacement implant is not an easy or straightforward process, and it comes with significant risk. Once the implant parts are removed, an antibiotic cement spacer is placed into the knee to keep the tissues at appropriate tension (to prevent

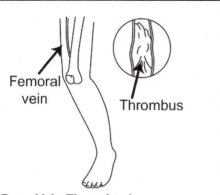

Deep Vein Thrombosis
Blood clots are among the more common complications following knee replacement surgery with potentially serious consequences. There are several methods to minimize this risk, though none are able to eliminate it completely. For this reason it is important to follow your surgeon's instructions closely.

excessive scar tissue formation, which would make putting new knee replacement parts in place nearly impossible). This spacer is not a functioning knee joint, and it is likely that you will be required to use a wheelchair during this time.

Daily injections of IV antibiotics will also be necessary, usually through a catheter/port placed into a vein in your arm. These antibiotics are chosen based on the specific type of infection a patient has. After four to six weeks of daily injections of antibiotics, most patients can expect an additional six to 12 weeks of antibiotics by mouth. Once this course has been completed, the patient will be held off of antibiotics for a period, to ensure that there is not any residual infection that has not been adequately treated. If infection does re-occur, then this process needs to be repeated.

Only once you have cleared the infection following "clean out" surgery and antibiotic treatments can you begin discussing replacing the knee implant with your surgeon. If you decide to move forward with another surgery, please be aware that revision knee replacement surgeries are not straightforward. Even with the spacer in place during the interim, tissues scar and bone loss occurs, making it more difficult for the surgeon to get the new knee implant in place.

Provided everything goes well with this revision procedure, the next step is intensive physical therapy. Physical therapy after a revision surgery can be extremely challenging given the enormity of the surgery, the patient's inactivity over the prior three to six months, and the affects that the infection itself had on the tissues. The expectations following this treatment course are extremely limited.

So how do we prevent infections from developing? The most obvious steps are all taken in and around surgery. These preventative measures include the clipping (not shaving) of hair around the surgery site prior to surgery, proper cleaning and preparation of the skin before surgery, and appropriate doses of antibiotics before, during, and after surgery, along with sterile techniques and the design of the operating room.

Patients can play a role in preventing infection, as well. Several steps that I recommend include washing your skin in the days leading up to surgery with a specialized soap, provided by your surgeon or the hospital, avoiding shaving your leg in the days leading up to surgery, maintaining a good diet following surgery, and meticulously caring for your wound until it completely heals without any further scabbing or drainage.

Infections are serious business, but they are very rare and significant attention is devoted to preventing them from happening. Infections occur in just 1% to 2% of knee replacement cases nationally. Given how rare it is for infections to occur after a total knee replacement, I would encourage you not to be scared away from the procedure out of fear of the potential complications.

Rather, I believe it's important for you to have as much information as possible in order to make an educated decision before having knee replacement surgery. With this information in hand, you will also be better prepared to do everything possible to minimize your risk of developing infection after your procedure.

3. Pneumonia

Pneumonia is another complication following surgery that is rare, but can have significant consequences. When this occurs, it is usually due to a combination of several factors.

The first of these factors is the type of anesthesia that you select. As detailed previously, when you have general anesthesia, there is the possibility that any stomach contents that you have, even if you were careful about not eating or drinking for eight hours prior to surgery, may be introduced into your lungs when the breathing tube is placed. This is very rare, but if it occurs, it almost always leads to pneumonia.

Other conditions that increase the risk for pneumonia following surgery are pain medications, which suppress the body's drive to breathe deeply, and relative inactivity, which also prevents the body from breathing deeply. When you do not breathe deeply, the small airways in the outer portions of the lungs can collapse, leading to blockage and fluid accumulation, which allows bacteria to grow and causes infection.

To prevent this, your surgeon and nursing team will provide you with

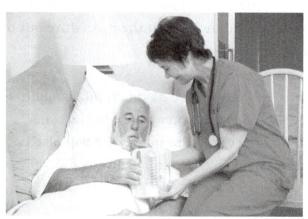 a device called an incentive spirometer, which encourages you to keep these small airways open. To be as effective as possible, the incentive spirometer should be used frequently, as often as every 10 minutes while awake. This

roughly corresponds to every commercial break during a TV program. Another method for breathing deeply is getting up and being mobile, which can stimulate deeper breathing.

4. Bedsores

Although bedsores are very rare after knee replacement surgery, they can have significant consequences when they occur. Bedsores are caused by inactivity and not shifting positions while sitting or lying.

While you are sitting in the same position, the blood flow to the skin you are sitting or lying on is cut off. If this happens for too long, the skin can die and begin to break down. When this occurs, the area has great difficulty healing and it becomes vulnerable to infection. Bedsores require very close attention and care, and oftentimes they involve further complications in the course of treatment. Having this wound increases the risk for infection following knee replacement. In the event that bacteria from the bedsores gain access to your bloodstream and make their way to your knee replacement, the results can be catastrophic.

5. Wound Healing Problems

This is another problem that is rare, but does put patients at significant risk for infection, and so I believe it is worth mentioning in this chapter. When a wound healing problem occurs, it is generally a situation where the patient has some underlying condition that impairs his or her ability to heal. The conditions that are most common in this scenario include inflammatory arthritis (rheumatoid, psoriatic, lupus), the medications used to treat inflammatory arthritis, as well as oral steroid medications, and diabetes, among others.

Most factors that increase the risk for wound healing problems are considered "modifiable" risk factors. These include smoking, obesity, and nutrition. Nutrition is important because if you do not have adequate building blocks to heal your wound, you will be unable to do so.

Smoking is particularly troublesome, as it attacks you in three separate ways that place you at risk for infection. This is not to mention the general health effects that smoking causes.

From an infection standpoint only, nicotine and the several other poisons found in tobacco smoke, impair the cells that form scar tissue and heal wounds. Tobacco smoke also decreases the blood supply and oxygen to the wound, and it impairs the immune system to the point where it is difficult to fight any infection if it does gain access to the wound.

Obesity has a similarly detrimental effect on wound healing. Adipose (fat) tissue has a relatively poor blood supply, preventing delivery of building blocks, and it tends to ooze fluid following surgery which keeps the wound open for longer, increasing the odds that something bad will find its way into the wound. Fat tissue is also rich in the nutrients that bacteria thrive on, making it a vulnerable environment to infection.

The best wound is one that is kept dry and covered until there is no longer any drainage and all areas are either completely healed or covered with stable, mature scabs.

You will either be sent home from surgery with a dressing that can stay in place until this occurs or with enough dressing supplies to accomplish this. If your wound continues to ooze or drain after returning home from surgery, or if you experience any increased redness, swelling, or pain in the skin around the incision, please inform your surgeon immediately for further evaluation and instruction.

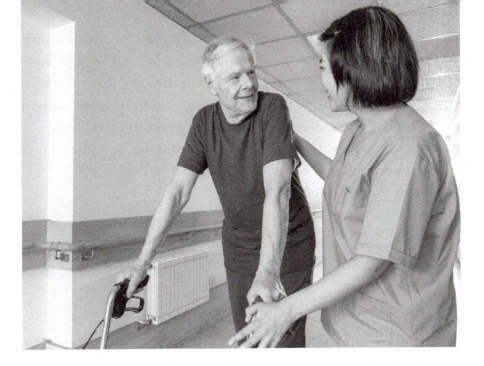

6. Falls

The risk of falling is increased after surgery, as your mobility is impaired and you will be taking pain medications. For these reasons, it is important that you take every step you can to decrease this risk.

As noted in previous chapters, clearing loose rugs, wires, and small furniture out of your recovery zone will help you navigate your home environment safely to prevent unnecessary falls. Some kind of anti-skid foot covering, such as no-skid socks, house slippers, or even shoes, is also a smart idea. Watch out for tight fitting coverings, though, as you will experience swelling in the foot on your operative leg and this may become uncomfortable.

Another time when falling becomes an issue is when patients are walking for rehabilitation and exercise after surgery. Rehabilitation should ideally be done in a controlled environment that is level and low in traffic. You don't want to have to dodge other pedestrians, or try and negotiate hills or rough terrain in your first few weeks following surgery.

I also recommend that my patients use a walker for the first month following surgery. I make this recommendation for two reasons. Firstly, using a walker slows you down so that you don't overexert yourself physically and set yourself back. Secondly, most patients have difficulty with balance and strength following total knee replacement surgery. If you do lose your balance, or you catch your foot on something, it is especially beneficial to have a walker available to prevent the fall.

Chapter 7
Maximizing Early Recovery

The hardest part of recovering from knee replacement surgery will come at the very beginning. From the moment you leave the hospital to approximately three months post-surgery can be a struggle, with significant pain from a large medical procedure. This is also the period where patients are required to work the hardest to regain knee motion.

The amount of work that's put in during these first three months will be evident for the rest of your life. Like the famous quote from Theodore Roosevelt goes, "Nothing in the world is worth having or worth doing unless it means effort, difficulty, pain..."

While this is the reality of the situation, there are several things that can be done to minimize discomfort and make the early recovery period as smooth and successful as possible.

First and foremost, I ask my patients to prepare themselves mentally for the challenges ahead. Realize that the early recovery period will not be fun, it will not be a walk in the park, and that it will require hard work and determination. But also, I want my patients to know that they will get through the early recovery period one way or another, and that the harder they work in the beginning, the happier they will be with the end result.

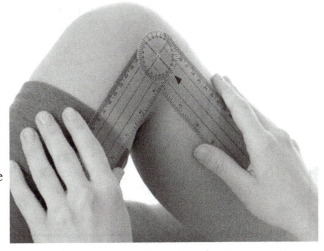

Physical Therapy

As previously mentioned, one of the most difficult parts of recovery is the physical therapy you are required to do following a painful surgery. Therapy is hard because you are in pain. But despite the fact that you are painful, you have to push through to achieve as much knee range of motion as possible.

Now you might say, why not wait until you have recovered to start therapy so that it is not so difficult? The problem is that you are in a race against the clock. This is due to the fact that considerable trauma is caused by the surgery itself, and your body will have to heal from that trauma. This healing is done through scar tissue formation, and scar tissue is inherently stiff. This is a problem, as a significant determinant in your satisfaction and function following knee replacement is how much knee motion you have.

To illustrate this point, you require at least 90 degrees of knee flexion (bend) to climb or descend stairs. If you don't achieve this goal by six to eight weeks following surgery, it is common practice to undergo an additional procedure, called a manipulation under anesthesia (MUA). During an MUA, you are put under anesthesia

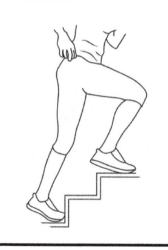

Why is knee motion so important?
Knee flexion is an important part of daily activities and certain levels are needed to perform basic tasks:

- *Level walking: 60 degrees*
- *Rising from a chair: 90 degrees*
- *Climbing stairs: 100 degrees*
- *Descending stairs: 100 degrees*
- *Tie shoes: 105 degrees*
- *Squat to pick up objects: 110 degrees*

Rowe, et al. 2000

and your knee is forcefully bent (with extreme care and caution) to break up scar tissue and allow increased motion of the knee. Although this is, thankfully, a rare occurrence, it does happen following 3% to 4% of knee replacement procedures.

To avoid this, it is important that you remain determined to gain as much knee motion as possible in the early weeks following your surgery. Physical therapy will play a major role in this process, and a qualified physical therapist is an essential part of post-surgery rehabilitation. While some jokingly refer to PT as "pain and torture" or "physical terrorism," it is important to realize that, while there is pain involved, this is pain towards a goal, and not for the sake of pain itself.

I have seen many patients who did not achieve their desired amount of knee motion on account of a poor relationship with their physical therapist, and they were ultimately left unsatisfied. Don't let this be you. If there is any indication that you do not work well with your therapist, be the squeaky wheel that gets the grease. Make your situation the best it can be to set yourself up for the most success possible.

Pain Control

While it is not realistic to expect that you will have no pain in the early goings following knee replacement surgery, or even once you are fully recovered, pain can be minimized with proper management.

The first strategy we have available for pain management is pre-medication. On the days of your therapy appointments, or even on your "off days" when you are doing exercises at home, I recommend timing your medications so that they are taking maximal effect while you are at physical therapy. There is some finesse to this, and it may take some trial and error before you get the timing exactly right.

As medications have side effects, based on how they affect you, you may have to balance your pre-medication delicately in order to maximize pain control and allow you to participate fully in therapy.

Another option is staggering medications. Your ability to stagger medications will be largely dependent on your surgeon's unique protocols. Staggering medications involves minimizing the time between doses of pain relievers.

Prescribed pain medications (opioids) are generally written to be taken only as needed, and only as often as every four to six hours. However, there may be times—such as during intense physical therapy sessions—when this may not be adequate to control the pain. During the time in between when you can take your prescription medications, you can take acetaminophen (generic Tylenol) or anti-inflammatories (which includes medications such as ibuprofen, naproxen, and meloxicam). These over-the-counter medications may not have the same level of affect that your prescription medication does, but they can certainly help bridge the gap until you can take your medication again.

Staggering medications may not be an option depending on some key aspects of your care. If you are on high power blood thinners following surgery, for example, then taking anti-inflammatory medications may not be allowed, as it may thin your blood too much. This may also be an issue if your surgeon sends you home with prescription pain medications with acetaminophen added in. Acetaminophen can be toxic to the liver in large doses. While this is generally not an issue when you taking it as needed for occasional aches and pains, it can be dangerous when it's used as an ongoing pain reliever. Therefore, if you are already getting acetaminophen in your prescribed pain medication, then you should not take any additional doses outside of this.

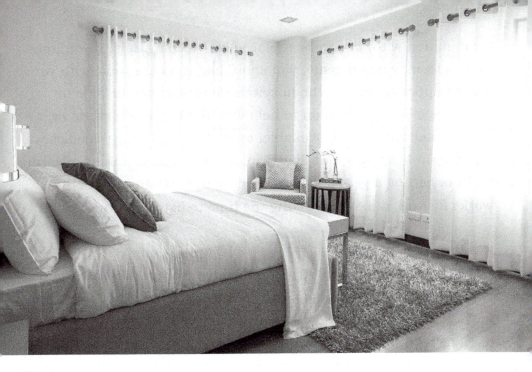

Sleep

Pain can impact people's sleeping habits, and not in a good way. Because pain tends to be worse at night, many patients who are in the early recovery process have difficulty sleeping.

You may be wondering why pain tends to be worse at night. The answer is simple. First, the knee tends to be more inflamed in the evenings, after a full day of activity and rehabilitation. Second, there are far fewer distractions at night to take your mind off of the pain, which makes it seem worse than it really is.

Sleep is a very important part of the recovery process. Lack of sleep can make you grumpy, less motivated, and it can decrease your ability to cope with the pain that you do have, which intensifies the situation. For these reasons, it is very important to find a way to maximize your sleep.

One of the best ways to get more rest during the early recovery period is by dosing pain medication before bed. This can be done in combination with, or can be replaced by, sleeping aids. If you know that sleep may be an issue, you should address the topic with your surgeon prior to leaving the hospital. He or she may be able to prescribe a safe medication to help with the process. Several over-the-counter options are available, as well as the home remedies we all grew up hearing about, like drinking warm milk, taking a warm bath, or getting a gentle massage before bed. Whatever it is that works for you, it is worth taking the time to figure it out.

Swelling

Swelling is very common during the early recovery period. Swelling is a significant cause of pain, due to the simple fact that your skin and tissues get stretched so much. Thankfully, we can minimize swelling with a number of techniques.

The best way to minimize swelling is with classic "RICE" therapy: rest, ice, compression, elevation. Try elevating the leg above your heart and use gravity to your advantage by encouraging fluid to return to your bloodstream. Compression works in a similar fashion, by physically forcing the fluid away from your knee, and preventing it from reaccumulating, as long as you are wearing the compression device. Ice limits the amount of fluid that accumulates creating swelling by causing the the blood vessels to shrink down in response to the cold temperature. When this occurs, there is more fluid that leaves the knee than accumulates, decreasing the swelling. Finally, rest can minimize swelling by decreasing the inflammation that causes swelling in the first place.

Skin Numbness & Tingling

Expect a fair amount of numbness around the outer portion of your knee in the weeks and months following surgery. The nerve branches that supply the outer aspect of the knee originate from the main nerve running on the inside of the thigh.

When the incision is made over the front portion of the knee, there is no way to avoid injuring these nerves. For some, numbness after surgery can be a permanent situation, however this is not common. For most, the nerves will begin to regrow in the early weeks and months following surgery and numbness will go away entirely by the end of the early recovery period.

As these nerves regrow, it is common to experience a tingling (pins and needles) and electrical sensation along the outer aspect of the knee. This can be uncomfortable at times, but it is a sign that things are continuing to progress, and it should only be temporary. As the nerves continue to grow, your sensation will begin to return to normal. This does not happen in a uniform fashion and some people will be left with small areas of permanent numbness.

Wound Care & Healing

Although we've talked about wound care and healing in previous chapters, I believe it's important enough to mention again, with specific regard to the early recovery period.

Active physical therapy is a necessary component of the recovery process, however all that bending and stretching does place stress on the incision site. If there are areas of weakness where healing is incomplete, then this may cause the incision to have small separations, which re-open the wound.

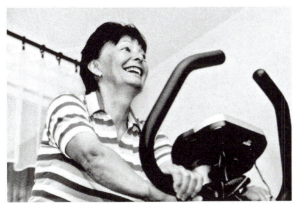

Physical therapy will help you regain strength.
This will occur through safe, everyday activities guided by your physical therapist to ensure you proceed safely.

These openings can drain, creating the opportunity for bacteria to gain access and cause infection.

Wound issues, which have been mentioned previously, should be addressed immediately. Although in many cases nothing needs to be done other than keeping the wound clean, dry and covered, there is a chance that further treatment may be necessary. Treatment for a wound infection may include anything from a short course of antibiotics by mouth, to being readmitted to the hospital for IV antibiotics, or even a surgery to clean out the wound and re-close it.

***

Complications following knee replacement are rare, and they get even less common the further you get from the surgery itself, but that doesn't mean that you should let your guard down. Remain cautious and always seek medical attention at the earliest sign of a problem.

Chapter 8
Transitioning to Mid-Recovery

With the first phase of recovery in the rear view mirror, things will really begin to look up. As you transition to the mid-recovery phase—from approximately three to six months post-surgery—you can expect to start feeling better and getting back to many of the activities you enjoy.

During the mid-recovery phase, you'll be developing a home exercise regimen and you'll slowly start returning to everyday activities, such as walking longer distances and even some recreational activities like golf and biking. Because your body has not fully recovered by the three month mark, it's important to keep up with all home exercise routines for the duration of the mid-recovery period. Muscles in and around the knee take a long time to rehab and build back up after surgery, and you will continue to experience minor discomforts and pain symptoms in the knee until you regain the full strength of your leg muscles.

Home Routines
An exercise program is something that you should have worked on and developed with your physical therapist before completing formal therapy. This should be a routine, and it should include a set of exercises that you are comfortable with. Routines that are too overwhelming or labor intensive are harder to maintain in the long-term. If you believe that your exercise program may fall into this category, please communicate with your physical therapist and work together to come up with a better routine.

Patient satisfaction after knee replacement surgery is largely tied to the strength of the quadriceps (quads), hamstrings, calf, and shin muscles. The most important of these are the quadriceps muscles, which are also some of the most difficult muscles to rehabilitate after surgery.

Quadriceps are difficult to rehabilitate for several reasons. First, the quad muscle is oftentimes weak even before heading into surgery. When one knee is painful, there is a tendency to rely more heavily on the non-injured knee, leaving the quad muscle on the injured limb to grow weak. Then, the quad muscles are injured during the surgery itself, and so for the first weeks following surgery the muscle continues to undergo a certain amount of atrophy. Because you use this muscle to stand and walk, you cannot overload your quads like you can your arms to speed the strengthening process. It takes a much more measured approach to build these muscles back up.

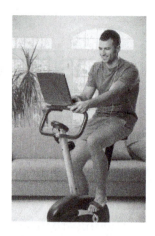

The Value of At-Home Exercise
The exercise you do at home plays an important part in the ultimate outcome of your knee replacement. This can also include even simple exercises, such as straight leg raises while you are watching television. I recommend that my patients do exercises during commercial breaks to help them with timing and repetitions.

Exercises

Several exercises can be used after knee replacement surgery, and it is best to work with your therapist to find a program that works for you. In this section, we will detail some of the more common exercises used and some concepts to minimize the inflammation and soreness that can arise from stressing your recently replaced knee.

1. Closed chain exercises: These are exercises where your foot is anchored to the ground or a solid platform. As your quads are not at full strength, and the motion is not completely normal, any motion at the knee will place additional stress on your ligaments and tendons. This is amplified by doing exercises where the foot is not anchored, such as leg extension exercises or hamstring curls. When the foot is firmly planted, it helps to stabilize the knee and minimize extra stresses placed on the knee. Most of the below exercises are "closed chain" exercises.

2. Isometric exercises: The knee is in an inflamed state while recovering from surgery. For this reason, additional motion through the knee, especially under increased loads of strengthening, can be damaging. To minimize additional motion, we have several exercises that strengthen the quad muscles without moving the knee joint. The two examples below—straight leg quad sets and wall sits—are of isometric exercises that will work to strengthen the quads while keeping the knee stationary.

Examples of Isometric Exercises:
•Straight leg quad sets: In a seated position, contract your quadriceps muscles to keep the knee locked straight, then raise the entire leg off of the bed/couch/floor so that your heel is above your hip. Repeat this 10 times, and do this every commercial break during a TV program.

•Wall sits: Place your back against a wall, place your feet shoulder width apart at a short distance from the wall, and squat down to a point where you are not comfortable, but not in obvious pain. Hold this position for 20 to 30 seconds, then rest. Repeat the series three to four times, and do this exercise three to four times each day. Depending on how you feel, you may want to modify how deeply you squat with each repetition. You should be able to complete three sets of 10 minute sessions

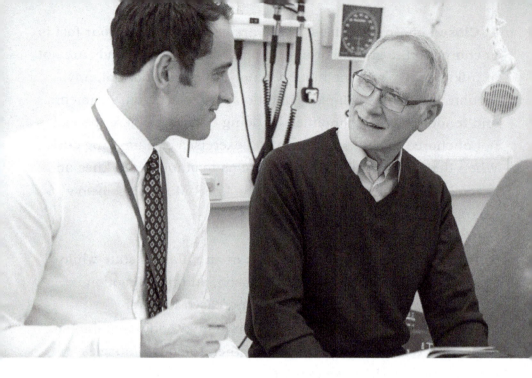

without extreme difficulty.

- Mini squats: Standing upright, with your feet shoulder width apart, squat down until you feel discomfort in your thighs, but again, not to the point of severe pain. Do this exercise with a chair in front of you or with a walker nearby, in case you need assistance. Do 10 squats and repeat the series two to three times. Depending on how you feel, you may want to modify how deeply you squat down with each repetition. You should be able to complete three sets of 10 reps in a five to 10 minute session without extreme difficulty.

- Modified lunges: Lunges are a great way isolate and build your quadricep muscle strength. These are easy to modify to fit your current strength level, depending on where you are at in the recovery process. When doing modified lunges, keep your feet shoulder width apart, hands on your waist, and step forward a comfortable distance, lowering your back leg toward the ground. Do not lower your leg too low, so that it is painful.

to a standing position. You can complete the recommended number of repetitions two ways. The first is to maintain one leg forward and complete 10 reps with the same leg. Another option is to alternate which leg you put forward until you complete 20 reps in total (10 for each leg). Repeat these three to four times per sitting and three to four times each day.

Quadriceps Strengtheners

For the reasons detailed above, quad strengthening is the part of recovery that can take up to, and sometimes longer than a complete year from surgery. That is not to say that you will be painful and unhappy this entire time. As I tell my patients, you will be 90% to 95% of the way to full recovery between three and six months following surgery. But because normal knee motion depends on a fully strengthened quad muscles, this leads to strain on the ligaments and tendons around the knee, which causes inflammation, soreness, clicking, popping, and swelling. As your quad muscles get stronger, these symptoms will be less frequent, and less severe. And even once you are fully recovered, they may not go away completely. But again, this should be rare, and you should feel significantly better than where you started.

As you strengthen these muscles between three months and one year, you will also notice that your confidence in your knee will improve, you will be more adventurous with your activities, and your endurance will increase, as well.

Returning to Activities

It is important to take a measured approach to activities, and explore your limits little by little. Before venturing out on a hike, or even a simple trip to the grocery store, make sure you are going to be able to make it back.

Patients will sometimes share stories about setting unrealistic goals as they recover from surgery, going to a mall for the first time, getting halfway through the trip and then realizing they are out of energy and their knee is in pain. I've heard stories of patients leaving full shopping carts in grocery stores when they realized they weren't going to be able to finish the trip and get everything home. When this happens, it can set people back for days, if not a week or two. An inflammatory flair can occur, and exercises become more difficult. This is why I recommend increasing your activities in small increments and not by leaps and bounds.

This also applies to getting back behind the steering wheel. While most people will be ready to return to driving during the early phase of recovery, it bears mentioning that the same incremental approach is recommended. Before getting in the driver's seat of a car, it's imperative that you are no longer taking prescription pain medications. You should also feel comfortable and physically capable of forcefully slamming on the brakes—imagine someone darting out in front of your car.

Before taking a real trip to a busy mall or grocery store, start by taking a practice run in an empty parking lot. See what it feels like to maneuver your leg into different positions. Try a few quick stops. Don't overdo it, but still try to get a sense for what it might be like if you were in certain situations. Once you feel comfortable in a parking lot, then try venturing out during times when traffic is minimal. You might also try driving on short trips, to familiar areas where you know your way around. Once you're able to navigate these areas with ease, then slowly expand your range.

Aches and pains are expected during the extended recovery period, but by this point pain control becomes an "as needed" situation, as opposed to the scheduled approach you likely required in the early phase of rehabilitation.

Anti-inflammatory medications are recommended here, as inflammation is often the source of pain. Blood thinning medications should be ceased by this point, so unless you have other reasons why you cannot take anti-inflammatories, they should be safe. If you are still on blood thinners, or there is another reason why anti-inflammatories are not recommended in your personal case, then acetaminophen can also be used.

Continuing to work hard throughout this phase of recovery will pay dividends. Your symptoms will be minimized, your confidence will be maximized, and you will be satisfied with your new knee.

Chapter 9

Increasing Strength During Late Recovery

Full recovery from knee replacement surgery can take up to one year, and sometimes even longer. Thankfully, the late recovery phase—which lasts from approximately six months to one year post-surgery—is usually the easiest phase of recovery. The governing principle during this phase is to increase activities incrementally, rather than diving in all at once.

All of the hard work you put in during the early and mid-recovery phases will be evident as the late recovery phase progresses, with increased comfort, strength, and endurance. It is very common for people to feel so good around this point that they accidentally overextend themselves. Don't make this mistake.

Overextending yourself during the late recovery phase, by taking on more than your body can handle, can lead to swelling, pain, and overall joint inflammation. While you are better equipped to deal with these issues during the late recovery phase than you were earlier on, too much stress on the joint can still lead to a downward spiral where recovery is interrupted. This interruption in strengthening can cause

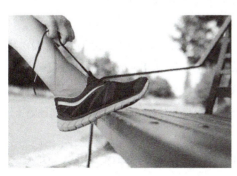

weakness, which makes motion and mechanics worse, increasing strain on the joint and causing more inflammation, starting a vicious cycle. For these reasons, I recommend avoiding overextending yourself, even once you feel fully recovered.

Some of the more common situations that can lead to overexertion during the late recovery phase include returning to golf, hiking, bike riding, and vacations. We will talk about many of these activities in more detail in following chapters.

As time goes by, your knee will begin to feel more "normal" and you may even forget that it was ever painful. As surgeons, we call this the "forgotten knee." It is the ideal goal when we perform surgery, because it means that the patient no longer considers his or her knee before doing activities.

It is completely normal to continue to have occasional aches and pains, swelling, redness, warmth, tenderness, and even clicking and popping during the late recovery phase, and even beyond that point. These issues will continue to decrease as your muscles get stronger and your knee motion becomes smoother, but they may continue even after a full recovery is complete. This typically happens when you are more active than usual, but can occasionally occur even when you have not done anything out of the ordinary. Aches and pains should be infrequent, and they should resolve in short order with minimal supportive care (rest, ice, compression, elevation, as needed anti-inflammatories.

You may be asking why anyone would go through this process only to continue having some of the same symptoms that led to surgery in the first place. It's a valid question. The answer is that the symptoms I've described should be orders of magnitude better than prior to surgery, and they should be much less frequent. While surgery may not eliminate every ache and pain around the knee, you can expect to feel light-years better after surgery than before.

Even with all the technology available today, it is impossible for a knee replacement implant to replicate the exact anatomy and mechanics of the human body.

As this is the case, we cannot realistically expect that a newly-replaced knee will feel like the knee you had when you were 18 years old. Instead, our goal is to improve your symptoms significantly, to the point where you can return to low impact activities without worrying that your knee will not support you.

If you keep this goal in mind and have realistic expectations of activities you want to return to, you will set yourself up for success.

***

Expect to return to the surgeon's office for repeat x-rays and an evaluation around one year after surgery. The most important aspect of this visit is how you are feeling and the trajectory of your symptoms. Unless you are having concerning symptoms, there is very little concern for implant complications after this point.

Not everyone feels 100% recovered a year after surgery. While that's not ideal, it's not something to worry about, either. As long as you are still seeing improvement, even if it is slow progress, you should expect to reach your goals eventually.

For those who have reached their full recovery, this is the beginning of a long-term maintenance program. Developing habits and routines will be one of the keys to keeping the strength and endurance that you have worked hard to gain over the past year. These same routines will keep your knee symptoms at a minimum going forward, as well.

Many people don't realize that knee health is a long-term endeavor until it's too late. If you cease participating in activities that keep your knee and leg strong, you can lose some of the knee motion and mechanics that you worked so hard to regain.

Inflammation, strain, swelling, clicking, popping, and even the sense of instability can all occur when patients fail to keep up with their long-term maintenance programs. If you continue with even a modest exercise and strengthening routine, you will significantly reduce your chances of these issues occurring.

Chapter 10
Debunking Common Myths

Many myths that persist regarding surgery, recovery, and long-term activities that you can or cannot do following knee replacement surgery. Let's take a look at the three most common and why they aren't true.

1. "During knee replacement surgery, the surgeon will cut out my knee joint and replace it with a large metal implant."

While there are relatively large metal and plastic implants used to replaced your joint surfaces, the term "joint replacement" is somewhat of a misnomer. One of the goals of surgery is to only remove the damaged tissues and bone, and maintain as much healthy bone and soft tissue structures as possible. For this reason, it would be better to refer to knee replacement as a re-surfacing procedure as this is truly what we are doing.

2. "After knee replacement I won't be able to kneel, or do other common activities of daily living."

While many people may find it uncomfortable to kneel after knee replacement surgery, this is strictly a patient comfort and self imposed limitation. There is nothing structural about knee replacement or surgery itself that would limit your ability to kneel on your operative knee. If you feel comfortable and can tolerate kneeling on your knee after replacement surgery, you are free to do so.

The same goes for most everyday activities following knee replacement surgery. You will find certain activities or motions may cause discomfort, but you are free to do what you feel comfortable with. The only exceptions to this are activities that require repetitive high impact motions, like jumping, jogging, and so on.

3. "My body will recover on its own, and physical therapy is just used to help speed this process along."

This is not only untrue, but a little dangerous. So much of your eventual happiness, function, and satisfaction with your knee replacement depends on the hard work and effort you put into your therapy in the early days, weeks, and months following surgery. This is because your body heals from surgery with scar tissue, which is inherently stiff. This scar will be mature by eight to 10 weeks following surgery, and when that occurs, whatever knee motion you have is what you will have forever. For this reason, you have to work the hardest in those first two to three months following surgery to gain as much motion as possible so that your knee functions properly and you do not end up with a stiff, painful knee joint.

Chapter 11

Protecting Your Investment

Considering all the time and energy that's gone into this process, you'll want to protect your new knee as much as possible. One of my mentors used to tell his patients to treat their knees like a fine piece of China. He was right. Protecting your investment is the key to making it last as long as possible.

The top three causes of revision in a knee replacement are infection, loosening of the implant, and knee instability, which can occur for several different reasons. The revision rate at 20 years out from surgery is about 10% of all knee replacements, but half of those revisions will happen within the first five years after surgery. Therefore, if you've already made it 10+ years with your new knee, the chances of needing a revision within the next decade are even lower than 10%.

While a certain numbers of revision cases are due to factors related to the surgery itself, many are not, and there are things that anyone can do to minimize the risk.

1. Infection As we have covered extensively in previous sections, infection after knee replacement surgery is a life changing event that should be avoided at all costs. We have already covered the steps you should take to minimize the risk, including using special soaps

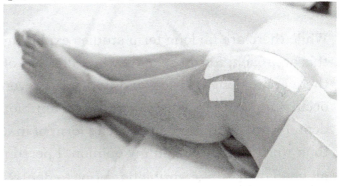

leading up to surgery, minimizing risk factors such as smoking, diabetes, and weight loss, and maximizing your diet with high protein and low carbohydrate foods. We have also covered the early-term strategies for minimizing the risk of infection, like keeping your wound clean and dry to help it heal as quickly as possible.

In the long term, and even once your wound is healed without scabs or other compromises in the skin, your risk of infection drops dramatically, but it never returns to the same low levels as non-replaced knees. With metal implants in your knee, if bacteria find their way into your bloodstream, they can find that metal and grab on. As the metal does not have a blood supply, your body cannot fight off infection once this happens. So once again, preventing this from happening is the best form of treatment.

Infection can occur in any number of scenarios, as there are many different ways for bacteria to find their way into your blood. One of the most common situations that we worry about is dental work. For this reason, some surgeons and dentists recommend taking antibiotics prior to dental work. This is a controversial area, and almost everyone you ask will have a different opinion on the matter. The American Academy of Orthopaedic Surgeons and the American Dental Association have concluded that this strategy is "cost effective" for the first two years following surgery.

While there are no long term studies exploring the effectiveness of this approach, for those of us who take care of patient infections, there are no lengths we would not go to prevent them from occurring. Taking a single dose of oral antibiotics one hour prior to dental work is an incredibly cheap form of insurance and more than worth the hassle, in my opinion. I personally recommend that all my patients take antibiotics prior to dental work indefinitely following knee replacement surgery.

Seeking prompt medical care, rather than waiting and watching to see if issues go away on their own, is another way to decrease the chances of an infection. The more you let things fester, the higher the likelihood that an infection finds its way into your blood and possibly to your knee. Get in to see your primary doctor or surgeon any time you have concern about infection. If you are concerned, your surgeon can make arrangements for you to be evaluated. These cases can be very serious, so please do not take no for an answer if your surgeon does not think your potential infection needs to be evaluated. Advocate for yourself and make sure that you get in to be seen as promptly as possible.

2. Implant Loosening Implants can be fixed to the bone in a few different ways. By far, the most common way to fix implants to bone is by using a polymethyl methacrylate polymer, or more simply, "bone cement." Bone cement is really more of a grout than a true cement. It bonds to the backside of the metal implant and presses into the nooks and crannies of the bone before hardening and grabbing hold. Bone cement generally creates a very tight bond, and it does not loosen even after decades of daily use.

In certain situations, however, this bond can become unstable and the implant can experience what is known as microscopic motion.

91

Microscopic motion is typically associated with very specific symptoms, such as pain that occurs with the first few steps. The pain typically will get better as you have been moving about, but then the pain will flare up again any time you temporarily take weight off of your knee—such as, when sitting down—and then stand up again to start walking. This is labeled "start up pain."

Start up pain tends to be very localized to the area of loosening, and it does not generally cause soreness of the entire knee. Having said that, when inflammation is serious enough, it may be difficult to pinpoint where this pain is coming from or say that it is limited to the first few steps after resting.

If this is the case, your surgeon will run a few tests to rule out infection. We check for infection first simply because of the dire consequences of missing an infection, as well as the fact that infection can present in any number of ways and mimic the symptoms of other conditions. Your surgeon may also order tests to look at the activity in your bone. This is called a three phase nuclear imaging bone scan, or more simply, a "bone scan." During a bone scan, a tracer material is injected into the blood, which will localize to areas of inflammation and bone activity. As implants which are loose stress the bone immensely, your bone will react vigorously, which causes a large amount of the tracer material to accumulate in the area. If microscopic motion is to blame for your pain, it will show up quite obviously on the bone scan.

As with so many other tests, there is the chance of a false positive during a bone scan. That is to say, a positive scan is only helpful in the setting of the correct symptoms. A negative scan on the other hand, is fairly definitive in showing that this is not what is causing your pain. If your scan is negative, then your surgeon should continue looking for an explanation for your pain.

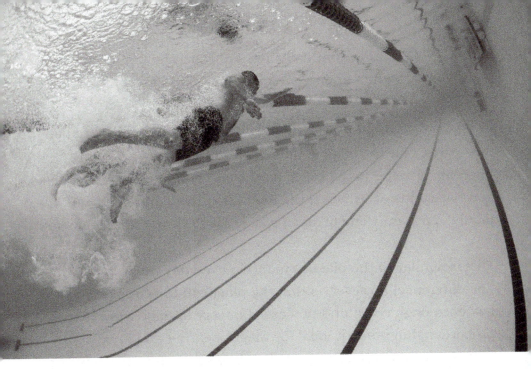

While surgical technique does play a role, there are a number of things that you can do personally to minimize your risk of implant loosening. The most important is to avoid repetitive high impact activities and stick to low impact exercises indefinitely following knee replacement. High impact activities include things like running, jogging, jumping, singles tennis, moguls skiing, basketball, and soccer. The repetitive pounding that occurs with high impact activities can have a mechanical effect to disrupt the microarchitecture of the bone and break up the bonds the cement has made. The other effect of this repetitive high impact activity, which can happen with loosening or in isolation, is accelerated polyethylene, or plastic wear. Stick to gentler activities like cycling, swimming, golf, hiking, and walking, and your new knee will thank you.

Even though high impact activities should be avoided on a repetitive basis, that doesn't mean you can never run or jog again. Your knee is strong enough to withstand these forces when kept to a minimum. If you are in a situation where your safety depends on your ability to run, RUN! But know that daily jogs are generally not a good idea for anyone who has undergone total knee replacement surgery.

3. Polyethylene Wear

Knee replacements are a combination of four parts. One is a plastic button on the joint surface of the kneecap, another is the metal on the end of the femur (thigh bone). You have a metal "tray" on the top of the tibia (shin bone), and finally, a polyethylene (plastic) spacer between the tibia and femur.

This is similar to the plastics found in everyday household items. The difference, however, is that the plastic in knee replacements has been engineered and processed in very specific ways to obtain properties that make it ideal for weight bearing and knee motion. To reiterate a sentiment detailed previously, as advanced as our engineers are today, nothing can replace what you were born with. With that being the case, the plastics used in knee replacements do not last forever. These are the weak link in your knee after surgery.

We expect that the plastic will wear out with time, though our goal —and your goal, too—should be to have it last as long as possible. Like the rubber in the tires of your car, the plastic in a knee replacement will wear down with use, and eventually it will need to be replaced. Our hope is that it will be 10, 15, or even 20 years before your knee replacement needs to be replaced. But much like the tires on a car, this is dependant on how much the knee is used. To continue with the car analogy, if you only drive 10,000 miles in a year, then your tires will last much longer than if you drive 100,000 miles in a year. The same goes for your knee.

A good example of this concept is the highly-advertised "30 Year Knee." The 30-year figure that is often touted in advertisements is based on laboratory studies showing that knee prostheses maintain reliable mechanics and function for 45 million simulated walking cycles. If you do the math, over a 30 year span, that averages out to just over 4,100 steps per day. Therefore, the more active patients are following knee replacement surgery, the faster this process will take place and the sooner a second, revision surgery will be required. With any revision surgery, the complexity is greater, and the risks for complications and inferior outcomes increase. As such, surgeons almost always recommend that patients do everything within their control to extend the lifespan of their knee implants.

Good research has shown that the younger a patient is when having knee replacement surgery, the higher the likelihood of someday needing a repeat surgery (Julin et al. 2010). This happens for a few reasons. The first is that people are living longer all the time, and this alone makes it more likely that someone who is young when he or she has knee replacement surgery will outlast the lifespan of the plastic liner. The other reason why younger patients are more likely to need revision surgery is because the younger a person is, the more he demands of his knee from a functional perspective. Younger people also tend to be more active, compared with the older population of people receiving knee replacements.

Chances are you're interested in knee replacement surgery precisely so that you can be active again. Do not despair. While we hope that your knee replacement lasts 15+ years, it is important that you remain aware of the limitations of your knee replacement and you continue to stay in contact with your surgeon for ongoing check-ups. Stay on top of it, even after surgery is complete, and make your knee a priority. It is standard for your surgeon to require that you return to clinic every one to two years after 10 years from surgery, just to monitor symptoms and the wear of your plastic. Issues that we catch early can be addressed with a much smaller procedure compared to issues caught in the later stages, once the entire knee has been damaged.

This applies to symptoms in your knee that you experience even before your surgeon wants you to follow up. Even if it has only been seven years since your knee replacement surgery, for example, you should still get evaluated if your knee becomes painful and the pain does not go away after a couple of weeks. If you have an infection somewhere else on your body, get it addressed right away. Make your knee, and your health in general, a priority.

Chapter 12
Sports & Exercise

One of the most common reasons why people pursue surgical treatment for their knee pain is to get back to the physical activities they can no longer enjoy. Golf, tennis, skiing, hiking, yoga, swimming, weight training, and so many other activities can be difficult—if not downright impossible—for adults suffering from debilitating knee pain. In this chapter, we will cover some of the most popular activities in-depth, including tips for enjoying these sports safely after knee replacement surgery.

Golf

More than 25 million Americans play golf each year, according to the National Golf Foundation, with seniors making up the lion's share of "core golfers" playing on a regular basis. Because of the stress that golf can place on the knees, it's not uncommon for golfers to come into my office looking for ways to ease their pain.

If you underwent knee replacement surgery with the goal of getting back out on the course, then you will have likely gone back to golfing in some form long before the late recovery phase (six months to one year). The following advice applies to the early goings of your return to golf, as well as during the late recovery phase, which is when most recreational players should return to the sport.

Having knee replacement surgery has been shown to increase your handicap. This is not true for hip replacement, however. It is unclear why this is, but is likely related to the different forces placed on the different joints. (Mallon and Callaghan 1992a) (Mallon and Callaghan 1992b)

Swing Adjustments

Most patients returning to golf after knee replacement will not need to make significant adjustments to their swings. If, however, a golfer's swing places a high degree of stress on his or her knee, then changes may be necessary.

- *Make sure your clubs are light and flexible. This can reduce strain on your knees and legs throughout your swing.*

- *Opening up your stance may relieve discomfort.*

- *Another common adjustment that golfers make following surgery is to switch to a walk-through or step-through follow through. This may put less strain on your knees.*

- *Decrease the swing plane in the direction of the impacted side to minimize stress on the joint.*

PGA champion golfer Gary Player has perfected these techniques, and his strategies can be seen in many online videos.

Golf can seem like a gentle alternative to more intense physical activities, however it is important to avoid jumping back in too quickly after knee replacement surgery. Slowly ease yourself back into the sport. Don't start with a competitive round of 18 holes while carrying your bag. In fact, I'd recommend not going directly back to the course at all. Start with working on specific aspects of your game, like your short game, which is considered the least physically demanding area of golf. Once you are feeling comfortable with this, slowly progress to chipping, and then make your way to the driving range. Again, start with the smallest bucket of balls and see how you feel. Be careful not to push too hard, as it will be easy to overdo it during your first few weeks back to the sport.

Consider wearing some type of support brace on your knee, as well. Your surgeon may have some specific recommendations based on your knee and surgery, but most over-the-counter braces should be more than adequate.

The golf swing places a significant amount of torque on the knee, so it will take some time to build up strength and comfort to handle this in a repetitive fashion. Avoid going back to the actual course until you've worked on your strength and you feel comfortable with the stress involved in playing this sport. If you take your time and don't rush it, you will be able to get back without too much discomfort.

Tennis

Tennis is another popular sport among the patients visiting me with knee pain issues. Unfortunately, tennis involves significant pounding on the knee joint. As we have covered previously, frequent pounding on the knee joint places patients at risk for implant loosening and accelerated wear, which makes tennis a high-risk activity following knee replacement surgery.

It's not just the running and jumping involved in tennis that makes the sport so difficult to return to after knee replacement surgery. It's also the pivoting and sudden change of direction that occurs, particularly with singles tennis. This places significant torque on the implant, as well as the remaining ligaments and tendons of the knee. Although implants are engineered to replace the portion of ligaments that have been removed in the knee, they are not designed to offer support at the high demands of pivoting and cutting sports, like tennis. When patients who have undergone knee replacement surgery do return to singles tennis, they place additional stress on the remaining natural ligaments to the knee, making them more prone to injury or even tearing.

Thankfully for tennis players, there is some good news here. While singles tennis is generally not recommended following knee replacement surgery, doubles tennis is much less demanding. Doubles tennis tends to involve less actual ground coverage and quick changes in direction, and for these reasons it is better on the knee replacement. Doubles tennis can be played after knee replacement surgery, provided you pre-warn your partner that you are not advised to aggressively pursue the ball.

Gentle, low-impact practice sessions with a partner, or with a ball machine, are generally safe after knee replacement, as well. As always, it is important to police yourself and not get carried away.

Skiing

Snow skiing is a great, low impact sport to enjoy after knee replacement. However, there are a few things to keep in mind when getting back to this activity.

Understand you are not going to be fully confident in your knee on your first few trips out, even if you have waited until you're fully recovered to return to the slopes. It is not likely that you focused on the muscle groups and motions involved in skiing in your rehab, so skiing is going to place new stresses on your knee. For these reasons, I recommend picking a day, or resort, where there are likely to be smaller crowds. This is a consideration even once you get comfortable again, because while you may be able to control yourself, you cannot control others around you on the ski hill, especially those who are just learning or those who lack a certain concern for the well-being of others.

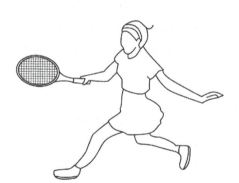

Doubles tennis is great sport to return to.
Doubles tennis minimizes the high impact and twisting movements, which you should avoid in singles tennis.

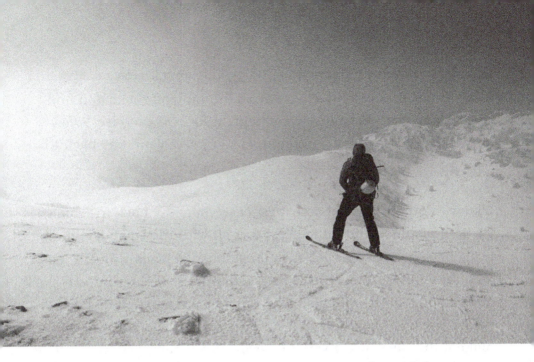

My next tip is to stick with well-groomed runs and avoid deep powder or highly technical runs (Black Diamonds).

While you may be confident in your knee and your skills on the slopes, there is a certain level of uncertainty with these types of runs that is impossible to eliminate completely. The last thing you want to do is get your ski or snowboard caught, which acts like a huge level arm, and twist or tweak your knee causing significant damage. Staying on groomed and prepared runs decreases your chances of running into trouble in these types of situations.

Finally, the last tip for returning to skiing, is to avoid large bumps and moguls. Not only are moguls bad for your other joints (ankles, hips, spine, etc.), but this type of repetitive, high impact activity may put you at risk for implant loosening and wear. It also puts you at increased risk of injuring your ligaments and tendons, as well, with the violent back and forth twisting that is required to appropriately navigate moguls.

Hiking

Hiking is a wonderful activity to enjoy following knee replacement. It is low impact (as long as you avoid jumping off rocks and find the path of least resistance), and a great form of exercise. A few important things to keep in mind as you make your way back to hiking:

Like with other physical activities, ease your way back in. This goes for both distance and difficulty. Start off with the least demanding trails first. Seek out paved or well-established trails with the least amount of physical obstacles as you gradually make your way back into hiking. You should also plan out your anticipated distance before any hike, knowing that however far out you get, you have to make it that far back. Even if it seems like a particular trail will be too easy, it's smart to err on the side of caution for the first few hikes after surgery. The last thing you want to do is get stuck out on a trail without the ability to get back.

Yoga/Pilates

Although yoga is not the first activity most people think of when they consider getting back into sports following knee replacement surgery, it is something that more and more people inquire about as they begin feeling better. Many people are surprised to hear that there are no restrictions to participating in yoga or Pilates following knee replacement surgery, as these activities do a fantastic job of encouraging flexibility and motion. The types of high-repetition, low-intensity exercises that are common in yoga and Pilates are great for building the foundational strength and endurance that helps people get the most out of knee replacement surgery.

Even though there are no specific positions or poses that are strictly prohibited based on the presence of a knee replacement, there may be poses that require modification, at least in the beginning. Make sure your instructor is aware of your knee replacement, and tell him or her where you're at in the recovery process prior to the beginning of class. Most instructors are able to accommodate students with physical limitations, particularly given how common knee pain has become.

Aerobics

Aerobics can be challenging following knee replacement, and it isn't something I recommend without first speaking to your physician. Many of the repetitive, high-impact motions associated with aerobic exercise are not a good idea following surgery, however there are still a number of options for maintaining your cardiovascular health. Safer alternatives to aerobics include swimming, power or speed walking, and the elliptical trainer. These activities are considerably lower-impact than aerobics, but they still provide ample benefits for your cardiovascular health.

If you belong to a gym or fitness center, look for group exercise classes with "low-impact" in the description. Low-impact classes should involve smooth motion at the knee joint without distinct periods of impact, which we know can accelerate plastic wear and put patients at risk of implant loosening. High-impact activities are not necessary for optimal cardiovascular health. In fact, low-impact activities like those mentioned above can get you to your desired heart rate goal, as recommended by the American Heart Association.

Swimming

Swimming is another great activity following knee replacement surgery. Not only does swimming boost cardiovascular health, but it is also a great way to build lean muscle mass, which can burn calories for you. Swimming regularly will also help stabilize your knee, helping it to function better in the long-term without relying on weight bearing or weight lifting exercises.

Water aerobics is another water-based activity that's great for building muscle without the added stress of gravity. Water aerobics is especially beneficial for those suffering from arthritis in other joints, which can make it painful to participate in land-based fitness classes.

One thing to be aware of is the downside of returning to swimming too soon after surgery. Ideally, your wounds should be completely sealed before getting back into the water. Even if areas of your wound have scabbed over and they aren't draining fluid, water can still loosen scabs and potentially re-open the wound. Swimming pool water will also serve as a conduit for the entry of bacteria into your wound, putting you at risk for infection at the surgical site. For this reason, most surgeons will discourage submerging your wound into the water, which includes both swimming pools as well as bath tubs. Individual surgeons have their own protocols as far as this is concerned, so I recommend discussing your desire to swim with your personal physician prior to getting into the pool.

Cycling

Cycling is not only good for the knee, it is also a great form of cardiovascular exercise. The key with getting back into cycling is to start out in a controlled environment without many cars or pedestrians.

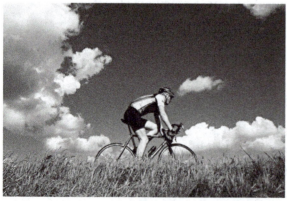

Begin cycling in a relatively flat area.
When done correctly, cycling is an activity that can aid in the recovery process after knee replacement surgery.

I recommend starting in a relatively flat area without too much geography (hills, valleys, etc.). Start off with a short distance and work your way up to longer distances only as you are comfortable.

One thing to consider as you begin cycling again after knee replacement surgery is the role that knee motion plays in your ability to operate a bike effectively. Until your motion improves, it will be difficult to bring your legs through a proper revolution of the wheels. To account for this, raise your bike seat. As your knee motion advances, you can gradually lower your seat until you reach your original position.

Cycling is an activity that can actually aid in the recovery process, if it's done correctly. To aid in the process of increasing your range of motion, try lowering your seat to just below where you feel comfortable. Continue working on this until you feel secure at this level, then repeat the process by lowering the seat some more. This should be done in a slow methodical manner, with days between each lowering of the seat, and not all in one sitting. Lowering a seat too suddenly could have deleterious effects.

Jogging/Running

As we have covered previously, I strongly recommend against jogging and running following knee replacement surgery. This is due to the increased risk of plastic wear and implant loosening. There are many other options for aerobic exercise that do not involve repetitive high impact activities, including water aerobics, power walking, the elliptical trainer, yoga, and cycling, to name just a few.

This is not to say that you will not be able to run after fully recovering from knee replacement surgery. Your implants and plastic are strong enough to withstand running in a situation where it is absolutely necessary.

If you find yourself in a dangerous situation and running will help get you out of that situation, run and don't think twice. But as far as regular exercise is concerned, running places far too great of a strain on the knee to be considered safe following surgery.

Weight Training

Many patients are surprised when I tell them that weight training is safe after surgery. In fact, there are no specific limitations on exercises or activities to avoid while weight training, outside of the same restrictions that have been repeated several times previously.

Of course, that doesn't mean I recommend returning to the gym and heading straight to the heaviest weights. High-impact activities are still a no-no, and your knee may feel better if you avoid open chain exercises or exercises that involve significant knee motion. Open chain exercises are those where the foot is not planted, or anchored to the floor or the exercise machine. In this position, the foot is loose, placing significant stress on the remaining natural ligaments of the knee (the MCL and LCL). Open chain exercises also place increased stress on the implants, as they are designed to replace two of the important ligaments of the knee (the ACL in all and PCL, in most designs). Exercises like seated leg extensions and prone hamstring curls should be avoided after surgery.

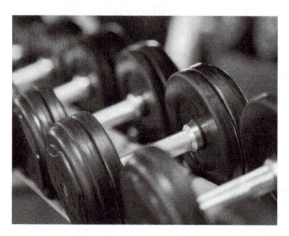

Weight lifting is safe to resume after knee replacement.
Strength training should be handled with caution. Ease your way back into this activity and ensure safety above all else.

On the other hand, isometric exercises can be an excellent option. Isometric exercises lock out the knee to minimize motion and isolate muscles around the knee for strengthening. Common isometric exercises include straight leg raises, quadriceps sets, and wall sits. Isometric exercises do not have to be the only type of exercise in your weight training routine, but can give your knee a break and help minimize the resulting inflammation if you mix them in among your other regular exercises.

Other Activities

There are many other sports and activities that knee replacement patients may want to return to, and some of these may require specific guidance or coaching. For the sake of brevity, I have tried to limit our discussion to the most common exercises that people ask about at my practice.

For specific instruction on the best ways to return to your desired sport, even the ones included above, seek out the advice of professionals in that area. Coaches and trainers should be able to come up with a personalized approach based on where you're at in the recovery process.

As a final note in this chapter, I want to repeat one more time just how important it is to ease your way back into physical activity, regardless of which specific activity you choose. Err on the side of caution, avoid or modify activities that require repetitive high-impact motions, and always stop as soon as you experience discomfort.

Chapter 13
Conclusion

Knee replacement surgery is extremely successful with a very high satisfaction rate. This is provided you have the right indication for having this surgery, are limited by your condition, and have the right expectations for your "new" knee following surgery and recovery.

Optimizing your health and nutrition leading up to surgery can go a long way in minimizing risk and decreasing the chances of possible complications during the recovery process. In fact, there are a number of things that you can do, both before and after surgery, to give yourself the greatest chances of a successful outcome. For example, simply being aware of the potential dangers following surgery and then working to minimize those dangers (as described in previous chapters) can make a big difference in your final outcome.

Recovery and rehabilitation after knee replacement are not easy.

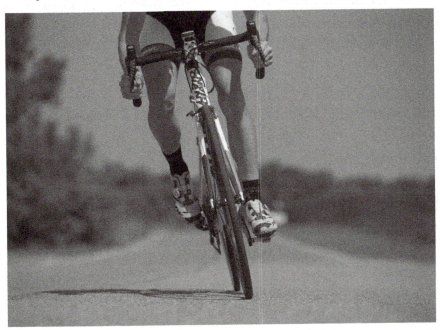

These steps require hard work and determination. But with your eye on the goal, and with the support of your surgeon, his team, and a physical therapist, you can expect a successful outcome. Even after a year-long recovery, it's still normal to experience clicking, popping, swelling, aching, and soreness in the knee with increased activity. This is expected, and it's not something to be overly concerned about. While you may never have the pain-free, perfectly-functioning knee that you had as an 18 year old, the final results from your knee replacement surgery should still put you in a significantly more comfortable place than where you began.

Finally, if you take anything from this book, I hope it is that caution is necessary whenever you're starting new activities following knee replacement surgery, regardless of what activities you're trying or how long it has been since your surgery. Be mindful of how to re-start physical activities and take the time to research potential modifications that may be necessary to keep yourself safe. While some of the most common sports and activities are covered in this book, I also recommend seeking out the advice of a professional in the area that you are interested in for more in-depth guidance.

Understand that no two people will have the same recovery process, and timelines for recovery after surgery should be taken with a grain of salt. It is very important to find a surgeon who you trust and feel comfortable with, and that you rely on this person to answer questions about your personal timeline and care. However, my goal with this guide was to offer readers a better understanding of the process leading up to, during, and following knee replacement surgery, and I hope that you feel more confident in your decision to explore this option after having read this book.

Chapter 14
FAQs

There are many questions that you will have leading up to and following surgery. Hopefully your surgeon and his team will address the majority of these before your surgery. The majority of joint replacement centers will also offer an instructional course that you will be required to attend prior to surgery.

Below are a list of the most frequently asked questions at my practice, however this is not meant to be an exhaustive list. Regardless of how prepared you are leading up to surgery, more questions will inevitably arise during the process. Write these questions down so that you can make sure to get them answered by your surgeon or a member of his or her team.

Q. HOW LONG WILL MY NEW KNEE LAST?

A. This depends largely on what you expect from your knee and how much you use it. Like the tires on a car, the more miles you put on your knee, the quicker it will wear out. With current plastics in the "average patient," we expect knee replacements to last greater than 10 to 15 years.

Q. WHAT IS THE RECOVERY TIME AFTER KNEE REPLACEMENT SURGERY?

A. This depends on your personal progress and pre-operative status. The overall recovery process can take over a year, but most patients are back to everyday activities between six weeks and 12 weeks after surgery, and they are 90 to 95% recovered between three and six months post-surgery.

Q. WHAT SHOULD I BE WORRIED ABOUT AFTER SURGERY

A. The most critical things to watch for after knee replacement surgery are infection, blood clots, and bleeding issues. Symptoms of these include:

- Increasing redness around the wound
- Increasing pain and swelling (It is normal to have increasing swelling and warmth following activity)
- A sustained temperature of more than 100.4
- Drainage from the incision
- Leg or foot pain and swelling that does not resolve with overnight elevation and use of compression stockings
- Bleeding gums or blood in the stool or urine

If these occur, call your surgeon's office or proceed directly to the nearest emergency room.

Q. HOW MUCH RANGE OF MOTION SHOULD I AIM TO ACHIEVE?

A. The more the better. It is generally accepted that you require 70 degrees of flexion to walk normally on level ground, 90 degrees to climb stairs, 100 degrees to go down stairs, and 105 degrees to get out of a low chair. To walk and stand efficiently, your knee should come within 10 degrees of being fully straight.

Q. WILL I NEED PHYSICAL THERAPY AFTER SURGERY?

A. Yes. This is perhaps the most important part of knee replacement. Physical therapy will begin almost immediately following surgery, and continue for six to eight weeks. This is where you will get all of the motion you can and work on strengthening your muscles to make your knee work properly. Expect to attend sessions one to three times per week. Keep in mind, though, that therapy is more about the work you do outside the office than it's about what happens in your one-hour sessions.

Q. DO I HAVE TO STAY AT A REHAB FACILITY AFTER SURGERY?

A. When at all possible, it is best for patients to return home after surgery. Even if you need to have family or friends fly to be with you, this is a better option than staying in a rehabilitation facility. In certain circumstances, however, it may be necessary to go to one of these facilities for a short stay, until you are safe to return home.

Q. WHEN DO I NEED TO FOLLOW UP WITH MY SURGEON?

A. Expect to see your surgeon, or a member of his team, two weeks after surgery to check your wound, pain, and progress in therapy. At six weeks, you'll be encouraged to return to the office for repeat imaging, and at 12 weeks for a final post-operative check. If you are doing very well at six weeks, your surgeon may choose to forgo the 12 week follow-up. On a longer term basis, expect to see your surgeon at the one year anniversary of your surgery. After this, follow ups are based on the surgeon's preference. Some surgeons choose to see patients yearly, others may wait until five to 10 years after surgery. If you ever have any issues or concerns, you should get in to be evaluated right away.

Q. HOW LONG WILL I NEED TO USE A WALKER OR CRUTCHES?

A. The general rule of thumb is that you need to use some kind of ambulatory aid until you can walk without a limp. Again, how long it takes to achieve this goal will largely depend on your personal progress with physical therapy.

Q. HOW LONG WILL I BE ON PAIN MEDICATION?

A. You will likely require some form of pain medicine, Tylenol or otherwise, for as long as three months following surgery. Strong pain medications (narcotics) are generally discontinued by patients by the six week mark following surgery.

With that being said, it's not uncommon that patients will continue to use these medications prior to therapy or prior to bed.

Q. HOW LONG WILL I BE ON BLOOD THINNERS?

A. You will generally be on some form of blood thinner for four to six weeks following surgery.

Q. HOW LONG DO I NEED A BANDAGE ON MY INCISION?

A. This will vary based on your surgeon's preference, but generally, once the incision is sealed to the point where there is no longer any spotting on the bandage, you can go without if you feel comfortable.

Q. WHEN WILL MY SUTURES OR STAPLES BE REMOVED?

A. It is rare that staples or external sutures are used in a first-time knee replacement surgery. Expect your stitches to be below the skin. They will dissolve over time, without needing to be removed. In the event that you do have an external closure device, it will come out at your two week follow-up appointment.

Q. WHY DOES THE SKIN AROUND MY KNEE FEEL NUMB?

A. It is normal for the skin around your knee to feel numb. The nerves that supply sensation to the leg come from the inside part of the knee and branch outward, and thus are cut when the incision is made for your surgery. This should improve with time.

Q. WHEN CAN I SHOWER OR GET THE INCISION WET?

A. This will depend on the technique and dressing type used by your surgeon. Oftentimes, it is OK to get the incision site wet after the first three to five days following surgery.

Q. WHEN CAN I IMMERSE MY KNEE COMPLETELY IN A BATHTUB OR SWIMMING POOL?

A. Your incision must be completely sealed, without any scabs present, before immersing your knee completely in any body of water.

Q. WHAT ACTIVITIES ARE PERMITTED FOLLOWING SURGERY?

A. In general, any low-impact activity is permitted following surgery. Only repetitive high-impact activities, such as tennis, jogging, basketball, and soccer, are discouraged. This is due to the effect on implant wear and potential implant loosening.

Q. WILL I BE ABLE TO CLIMB AND DESCEND STAIRS AFTER KNEE REPLACEMENT SURGERY?

A. Prior to leaving the hospital, you will work with physical therapy on going up and down stairs. If you have stairs in your home, you will want to avoid using these on a regular basis, and you should work to arrange your recovery zone downstairs.

Q. HOW MUCH WEIGHT CAN I PLACE ON MY KNEE AFTER SURGERY?

A. In a "straightforward" surgery, you should be able to place full weight on your knee immediately following surgery. If there are any uncommon aspects to your situation, be sure to discuss this question with your surgeon, as the answer may vary depending on the quality of your bone and any abnormalities in your anatomy.

Q. CAN I KNEEL AFTER SURGERY?

A. Once your incision is healed, it is up to you. Whether or not you kneel should be based on your comfort level.

You will not damage your knee by kneeling, but you may not like how it feels.

Q. WHEN CAN I RETURN TO WORK?

A. This will depend on your line of work and your comfort after surgery. If there is light duty available, or if you have a stationary job, then you can most likely return to work within four to six weeks after surgery. If your job is more strenuous and requires significant time on your feet, expect to be away for as long as eight to 12 weeks.

Q. WHEN CAN I RESUME PHYSICAL ACTIVITIES?

A. Expect to be up and walking around as much as you feel comfortable as soon as you leave the hospital. Be careful not to overdo it. In terms of other activities, these will be based on your progress and pain control in association with your surgeon.

Q. CAN I USE WEIGHTS WHEN I EXERCISE?

A. It is unlikely that you will want to use weights in the first one to two months following surgery. After this, when you are feeling more comfortable, it is OK to start using weights in a graduated fashion, starting with low weight and working your way up slowly.

Q. CAN I RETURN TO DOWNHILL SKIING?

A. Skiing is a low impact activity that will not damage your knee. There is risk, however, from the potential of falling or crashing. You should not resume moguls skiing after knee replacement as this is high impact and can damage the components of your knee implant.

Q. WHEN CAN I RESUME SEXUAL ACTIVITY?

A. This will largely depend on your comfort level, but most people can resume sexual activities within four to six weeks following surgery.

Q. ARE THERE POSITIONS FOR SITTING OR SLEEPING THAT I CANNOT BE IN?

A. There are no restrictions on the position of your knee. Based on your progress with therapy in achieving the desired knee range of motion, your therapist may recommend positions to help you make progress. Otherwise, this should be guided by comfort.

Q. WHEN CAN I DRIVE?

A. This depends on two things. First, you must be no longer taking narcotic pain medication. Second, you must feel confident in your ability to slam on the brakes without hesitation, were it necessary to do so. That being said, many surgeons have varying opinions on this matter. Please check with your surgeon.

Q. WHEN CAN I TRAVEL?

A. This is somewhat of a controversial topic, but typically you can travel by airplane or car whenever you feel comfortable doing so. Make sure to walk every hour or two to stretch your legs and keep blood flowing while you are en route to your destination.

Q. CAN I DRINK ALCOHOL DURING MY RECOVERY?

A. Alcohol should be avoided for as long as you are on strong pain medications or blood thinners, as it can intensify the effects of both.

Q. WHAT ARE GOOD AND BAD POSITIONS FOR MY KNEE DURING RECOVERY?

A. Good positions are ones that promote full extension (straightening) and deep flexion (bending) of the knee. Bad positions are ones that keep your knee slightly bent (a pillow under the knee).

Q. SHOULD I APPLY ICE OR HEAT AFTER SURGERY?

A. Ice is best at first because it can help minimize inflammation and swelling. After the first few weeks, it is up to you whether you decide to apply ice or heat to your knee, depending on whether the application provides you with any comfort.

Q. HOW LONG SHOULD I WEAR COMPRESSION STOCKINGS?

A. Some surgeons do not have their patients use stockings after knee replacement surgery. If your surgeon does, ask him what he recommends. Generally speaking, you should wear compression stockings until your swelling is back to what it was prior to surgery.

Q. WHAT SHOULD I DO IF I'M CONSTIPATED?

A. Constipation is expected following knee replacement surgery due to medications, anesthesia, and decreased mobility. You should leave the hospital with prescriptions for stool softeners. If not, proceed to the drug store for some as soon as possible. Staying well hydrated and eating plenty of fiber can minimize the effects, as well.

Q. WHAT CAN I DO ABOUT INSOMNIA AFTER SURGERY?

A. Insomnia is common following knee replacement surgery. Again, this can be due to several factors, such as anesthesia, medications, inability to be active during the day. Over-the-counter medications, such as Benadryl, melatonin, Tylenol PM, may be effective. Insomnia generally gets better with time. If it continues to be a problem, contact your primary care physician.

Q. WHAT RANGE OF MOTION SHOULD I EXPECT FROM MY KNEE AFTER ONE YEAR?

A. You should hopefully be very close to your full range of motion by six weeks after surgery. You will likely make minor additional gains following this as long as you continue to work on it. In general, it has been shown that your final range of motion will likely fall within 10 degrees of where you started.

Q. DO I NEED ANTIBIOTICS BEFORE HAVING DENTAL WORK OR OTHER INVASIVE MEDICAL PROCEDURES?

A. This is a very controversial topic. Most surgeons recommend antibiotics before dental work for the first two years after surgery. Some will say indefinitely. Ask your surgeon for his or her opinion on the matter.

Q. WILL MY KNEE SET OFF METAL DETECTORS AT THE AIRPORT?

A. Likely so. This will depend on the sensitivity of the detector, but most will be set off. You may be required to show your scar and undergo wand screening.

Q. WHAT SHOULD I KNOW ABOUT COMPUTER-ASSISTED SURGERY?

A. Computer-assisted surgery is an exciting new area of joint replacement, however it is still developmental at this time. Computer-assisted surgery does not have a proven track record, even though it does have the potential to be a useful tool in performing an already very successful operation.

Specifically, computer-assisted surgery can be useful in the setting of altered anatomy or prior knee surgery that would preclude the use of standard instrumentation. For further information regarding computer-assisted surgery, please see the American Association of Hip and Knee Surgeons Position Statement on computer-assisted surgery at: http://www.aahks.org/pdf/CAOSpositionstatement.pdf

Q. WILL I NEED A CPM (CONTINUOUS PASSIVE MOTION) MACHINE?

A. This is an area of mild controversy. While some surgeons still use this device, there is little evidence to show that it makes any difference in long term outcomes following knee replacement surgery. There is even some evidence that CPM machines may negatively impact surgical outcomes by giving patients a false sense of progress, when little or none is actually being made.

Q. IS THERE A ROLE FOR "MIS" (MINIMALLY INVASIVE SURGERY/ MINIMAL INCISION SURGERY)?

A. In general, surgeons use the smallest incision necessary to do the job correctly. It is not worth risking long term issues because of improper techniques in the name of using a smaller incision. Further information regarding MIS surgery is best obtained from the American Association of Hip and Knee Surgeons Position Statement on MIS surgery. For further information, please visit http:// www.aahks.org/pdf/MIS_Patients.pdf

Q. I THINK MY LEG FEELS LONGER NOW. IS THIS POSSIBLE?

A. It is not uncommon to have this sensation following surgery. While rare to have an actual change in leg length, the sensation is often due to muscles and tendons adjusting to a new situation. In rare cases, patients who started with severe deformities before surgery may end up with a leg getting longer once it is made straight again.

Q. MY KNEE MAKES AN INTERMITTENT CLICKING OR POPPING NOISE. IS THIS NORMAL?

A. This is completely normal. The noise you are hearing is the plastic and metal contacting each other. This should decrease with time as you will form scar tissue covering some of these surfaces, and as your muscle strength improves making your knee motion more smooth, but it will likely persist at some level indefinitely.

Q. CAN I GET AN MRI WITH A KNEE REPLACEMENT?

A. Yes. The metal in the knee replacement may alter the images of tissues immediately around the knee, but it will have no effect on imaging of tissues away from the knee.

Q. WHAT ARE MY CHANCES OF A SUCCESSFUL OUTCOME?

A. Success is defined in several different ways. For my patients, I will ask the following questions:

- Are you glad you had the operation?
- Were your expectations realistic and were they met?
- Would you do it again?

Based on the literature, approximately 90% to 95% of knee replacement patients answer yes to all three of these questions at one year after surgery.

Chapter 15
References

For more information on all aspects of total hip replacement surgery, please visit the website for the American Academy of Orthopaedic Surgeons (AAOS). There, you'll find articles, diagrams, and videos describing the entire process. Below, is a list of references cited within this book.

Barad, Steven J., Stephen M. Howell, and Tom Joyce. 2015. "Is a Shortened Length of Stay and Increased Rate of Discharge to Home Associated with a Low Readmission Rate and Cost-Effectiveness after Primary Total Knee Arthroplasty?" Arthroplasty Today. doi:10.1016/j.artd.2015.08.003.

Culliton, Sharon E., Dianne M. Bryant, Tom J. Overend, Steven J. MacDonald, and Bert M. Chesworth. 2012. "The Relationship between Expectations and Satisfaction in Patients Undergoing Primary Total Knee Arthroplasty." The Journal of Arthroplasty 27 (3): 490–92.

da Costa, Bruno R., Eveline Nüesch, Rahel Kasteler, Elaine Husni, Vivian Welch, Anne W. S. Rutjes, and Peter Jüni. 2014. "Oral or Transdermal Opioids for Osteoarthritis of the Knee or Hip." Cochrane Database of Systematic Reviews , no. 9 (September): CD003115.

Deyle, G. D., N. E. Henderson, R. L. Matekel, M. G. Ryder, M. B. Garber, and S. C. Allison. 2000. "Effectiveness of Manual Physical Therapy and Exercise in Osteoarthritis of the Knee. A Randomized, Controlled Trial." Annals of Internal Medicine 132 (3): 173–81.

Hootman, Jennifer M., Charles G. Helmick, Kamil E. Barbour, Kristina A. Theis, and Michael A. Boring. 2016. "Updated Projected Prevalence of Self-Reported Doctor-Diagnosed Arthritis and Arthritis-Attributable Activity Limitation Among US Adults, 2015-2040." Arthritis & Rheumatology (Hoboken, N.J.) 68 (7): 1582–87.

Horlocker, Terese T., Sandra L. Kopp, Mark W. Pagnano, and James R. Hebl. 2006. "Analgesia for Total Hip and Knee Arthroplasty: A Multimodal Pathway Featuring Peripheral Nerve Block." The Journal of the American Academy of Orthopaedic Surgeons 14 (3): 126–35.

"Information Statement." 2016. Accessed June 27. http:// www.aaos.org/CustomTemplates/Content.aspx?id=5593. Keswani, Aakash, Michael C. Tasi, Adam Fields, Andrew J. Lovy, Calin S. Moucha, and Kevin J. Bozic. 2016. "Discharge Destination After Total Joint Arthroplasty: An Analysis of Postdischarge Outcomes, Placement Risk Factors, and Recent Trends." The Journal of Arthroplasty 31 (6): 1155–62.

Keswani, Aakash, Mitchell C. Weiser, John Shin, Andrew J. Lovy, and Calin S. Moucha. 2016. "Discharge Destination After Revision Total Joint Arthroplasty: An Analysis of Postdischarge Outcomes and Placement Risk Factors." The Journal of Arthroplasty 31 (9): 1866–72.e1.

Mallon, W. J., and J. J. Callaghan. 1992a. "Total Hip Arthroplasty in Active Golfers." The Journal of Arthroplasty 7 Suppl: 339–46. 1992b. "Total Hip Arthroplasty in Active Golfers." The Journal of Arthroplasty 7 Suppl: 339–46.

Noble, Philip C., Michael A. Conditt, Karon F. Cook, and Kenneth B. Mathis. 2006. "The John Insall Award: Patient Expectations Affect Satisfaction with Total Knee Arthroplasty." Clinical Orthopaedics and Related Research 452: 35–43.

Núñez, Montserrat, Núñez Montserrat, Lozano Luis, Núñez Esther, Josep M. Segur, Sastre Sergi, Maculé Francisco, Ortega Raquel, and Suso Santiago. 2009. "Total Knee Replacement and Health-Related Quality of Life: Factors Influencing Long-Term Outcomes." Arthritis & Rheumatism 61 (8): 1062–69.

Ritter, Merrill A., Michael E. Berend, Leesa D. Harty, Kenneth E. Davis, John B. Meding, and E. Michael Keating. 2004. "Predicting Range of Motion after Revision Total Knee Arthroplasty: Clustering and Log-Linear Regression Analyses." The Journal of Arthroplasty 19 (3): 338–43.

Rowe, PJ, Myles, CM, Walker, C, Nutton, R, Knee joint kinematics in gait and other functional activities measured using flexible electrogoniometry: how much knee motion is sufficient for normal daily life. Gait & Posture. 12(2): 143-155

Skoffer, Birgit, Thomas Maribo, Inger Mechlenburg, Per M. Hansen, Kjeld Søballe, and Ulrik Dalgas. 2016. "Efficacy of Preoperative Progressive Resistance Training on Postoperative Outcomes in Patients Undergoing Total Knee Arthroplasty." Arthritis Care & Research 68 (9): 1239–51.

Walls, Jason D., Daniel Abraham, Charles L. Nelson, Atul F. Kamath, Nabil M. Elkassabany, and Jiabin Liu. 2015. "Hypoalbuminemia More Than Morbid Obesity Is an Independent Predictor of Complications After Total Hip Arthroplasty." The Journal of Arthroplasty 30 (12): 2290–95.

Wisse, B. E. 2004. "The Inflammatory Syndrome: The Role of Adipose Tissue Cytokines in Metabolic Disorders Linked to Obesity." Journal of the American Society of Nephrology: JASN 15 (11): 2792–2800.